Epidemiology Step by Step

Mastering the Fundamentals of Disease Tracking and Control

David Merrill

PREFACE

Welcome to *Epidemiology Step by Step*. This book was designed with you in mind—whether you're new to the field of epidemiology, a student looking to solidify your understanding, or a professional wanting a clear and structured guide to core concepts. Epidemiology is often referred to as the cornerstone of public health, and for good reason. It's the science that allows us to understand how diseases spread, who is most affected, and what we can do to prevent and control these health threats.

When I first became interested in epidemiology, I was struck by its ability to connect science, policy, and real-world impact. It provides the concepts and frameworks we need to identify health issues in communities, track the spread of infectious diseases, and address chronic conditions that impact millions of people around the world. But I also noticed that the field can seem complex and daunting to newcomers, with many technical terms and study designs to navigate. That's why I decided to write this book in a way that breaks down the fundamental concepts, making them easy to understand without losing any depth.

Why This Book?

There are many textbooks and resources on epidemiology, but many of them are either too technical or too focused on specific areas. What I wanted to create was a comprehensive yet approachable guide that walks you through the key topics in a logical sequence. Each chapter builds on the previous one, helping you see the bigger picture and how different parts of epidemiology fit together.

This book covers everything from the foundational principles to advanced topics like genetic epidemiology and the impact of big data on disease tracking. You'll learn how epidemiologists study health at the population level, how they investigate outbreaks, and how they identify the causes of chronic diseases like cancer and diabetes. Along the way, you'll also gain an understanding of the tools and techniques epidemiologists use to collect, analyze, and interpret data.

The first chapter offers a broad introduction, laying the groundwork by explaining what epidemiology is, its history, and why it has such an important role in public health. After that, we go into the specifics—like how to measure disease frequency, the different types of study designs used in epidemiology, and how to interpret the risk of disease. By the time you reach the later chapters, you'll be ready to tackle more advanced topics, such as the influence of genetics and environmental factors on health.

Who Is This Book For?

This book is for anyone with an interest in understanding the science behind how diseases affect populations and what can be done to prevent them. It's especially useful for:

- **Students**: Whether you're studying public health, biology, or a related field, this book will help you build a strong foundation in epidemiology. Each chapter introduces new concepts in a clear and structured way, with real-world examples to illustrate key points.
- **Healthcare professionals**: If you're a doctor, nurse, or public health worker, this book will give you a deeper understanding of how the data you encounter in your daily work fits into the larger context of population health. You'll learn how to interpret disease trends, assess risk factors, and apply epidemiological principles to improve patient outcomes.
- **Anyone interested in public health**: If you've ever wondered how we track outbreaks, why certain diseases spread in particular ways, or how we determine the effectiveness of vaccines, this book will provide the answers. Even if you don't have a scientific background, the concepts are explained in simple, accessible language that anyone can follow.

What You Can Expect

The book is divided into 17 chapters, each focusing on a specific area of epidemiology. In Chapter 1, we start with the basics—defining epidemiology, exploring its history, and understanding its role in public health. From there, we move into more detailed topics:

- **Measuring disease frequency** (Chapter 2) teaches you how to calculate key metrics like incidence and prevalence, which are critical for understanding how common diseases are in different populations.
- **Study designs** (Chapter 3) shows you the different ways epidemiologists investigate health issues, from observational studies to case-control and cohort studies. This chapter also explains the strengths and limitations of each method.
- **Outbreak investigation** (Chapter 6) walks you through the steps epidemiologists take to identify the source of an outbreak and contain it before it spreads further. You'll learn about famous cases like the cholera outbreak in London that led to the birth of modern epidemiology.
- **Bias and confounding** (Chapter 8) explains the challenges epidemiologists face in ensuring their results are accurate and reliable, and how they control for factors that could skew their findings.

The final chapters cover emerging topics in epidemiology, including the role of **genetic factors** in health (Chapter 14), **global health** challenges (Chapter 15), and how **big data** and **artificial intelligence** are changing the way we track and respond to diseases (Chapter 16).

A Step-by-Step Approach

Throughout the book, I've aimed to take a step-by-step approach that builds your knowledge progressively. You'll start with basic concepts and gradually move into more complex areas, always with clear explanations and practical examples. My goal is for you to come away from this book not just with knowledge but with the confidence to apply epidemiological principles in the real world.

Thank you for picking up *Epidemiology Step by Step*. I hope it helps you discover the exciting and impactful field of epidemiology and inspires you to think about how we can improve public health through science and data.

TOPICAL OUTLINE

Chapter 1: Introduction to Epidemiology
- Definition and Scope of Epidemiology
- History and Evolution of Epidemiology
- Key Roles of an Epidemiologist
- Health and Disease: Basic Concepts
- Population vs. Individual Health Perspectives
- The Epidemiologic Triangle: Host, Agent, Environment
- Epidemiology's Role in Public Health Policy
- Understanding Disease Distribution: Time, Place, and Person
- Key Metrics: Morbidity, Mortality, and Risk
- How Epidemiology Informs Public Health Interventions

Chapter 2: Measures of Disease Frequency
- Incidence and Prevalence
- Person-Time Measures
- Standardized Rates and Ratios
- Adjusting for Age and Other Demographic Factors

Chapter 3: Study Designs in Epidemiology
- Observational vs. Experimental Studies
- Cross-Sectional Studies
- Cohort Studies
- Case-Control Studies
- Nested Case-Control and Case-Cohort Studies

Chapter 4: Measuring and Interpreting Risk
- Absolute vs. Relative Risk
- Odds Ratio and Risk Ratio
- Attributable Risk
- Number Needed to Treat (NNT) and Number Needed to Harm (NNH)

Chapter 13: Social Determinants of Health in Epidemiology
- Socioeconomic Status and Health Disparities
- Impact of Race, Ethnicity, and Gender on Health Outcomes
- The Role of Education and Employment in Health

Chapter 14: Genetic Epidemiology
- Heritability and Genetic Risk Factors for Disease
- Gene-Environment Interactions
- Population Genetics in Epidemiologic Studies

Chapter 15: Epidemiology and Global Health
- Emerging and Re-Emerging Infectious Diseases
- Global Surveillance Systems (WHO, CDC, etc.)
- Epidemiology of Pandemics: Historical and Modern Examples
- Vaccination Programs and Disease Eradication

Chapter 16: Future Trends and Challenges in Epidemiology
- Big Data and Epidemiology: Opportunities and Challenges
- The Role of Artificial Intelligence in Disease Surveillance
- Climate Change and Its Impact on Disease Patterns

Chapter 17: History and Terms
- History of Epidemiology
- Terms and Definitions

Afterword

TABLE OF CONTENTS

CHAPTER 1: INTRODUCTION TO EPIDEMIOLOGY

Definition and Scope of Epidemiology

Epidemiology is the study of how diseases spread, who gets them, and why. It helps us understand the patterns and causes of health problems in populations, not just individuals. At its core, **epidemiology looks at the frequency, distribution, and determinants of disease**. Frequency refers to how often a disease occurs. This can be measured through incidence, the number of new cases within a specified time, and prevalence, the total number of cases at a particular time. Both are vital for understanding how widespread a disease is and how quickly it's spreading.

The scope of epidemiology extends beyond just infectious diseases. It covers any health-related conditions, including chronic diseases like diabetes and heart disease, injuries, and environmental exposures, such as air pollution or toxic substances. By analyzing these events, epidemiologists can pinpoint factors that increase the risk of health problems. For example, they might investigate how smoking contributes to lung cancer or how obesity relates to heart disease. The information gathered allows us to prevent and control disease outbreaks or improve health outcomes.

Epidemiology involves several key concepts that guide its practice. One of the primary ideas is **population**. Unlike clinical medicine, which focuses on individuals, epidemiology focuses on groups of people. These groups might be defined by geography, demographics, behavior, or other factors. This population-based approach helps identify trends and causes that wouldn't be apparent if only individual cases were studied.

Another critical concept in epidemiology is **comparison**. Epidemiologists often compare different populations or groups within the same population to find patterns. For example, they might compare smokers with non-smokers to see how their risks for certain diseases differ. This comparative method is key in identifying the factors that contribute to disease risk and progression.

Causality is another essential aspect of epidemiology. Establishing what causes a disease is not always straightforward. Often, there are multiple factors involved. Epidemiologists use various study designs to identify these causes, including observational studies (like cohort or case-control studies) and experimental studies (such as randomized controlled trials). These methods help build evidence on the relationships between exposures (like pathogens or lifestyle choices) and outcomes (such as illnesses).

Epidemiologists also rely heavily on **data collection and analysis**. Data comes from a variety of sources, including health surveys, medical records, and laboratory tests. Once data is collected, it's analyzed to detect patterns and make predictions about future disease trends. For example, they might look at how often a flu outbreak occurs in a community and project the likelihood of another outbreak happening soon.

In addition, **epidemiology considers risk factors**. Risk factors are elements that increase the likelihood of developing a disease. These can be biological (like genetics), behavioral (such as physical activity levels), or environmental (like air quality). Identifying these risk factors allows epidemiologists to propose interventions or policies aimed at reducing exposure or mitigating their effects.

A critical area of epidemiology is **surveillance**. This involves the ongoing collection and analysis of health data to track disease trends over time. Surveillance systems monitor diseases and other health-related events, providing valuable information for early warning systems. For instance, the detection of an unusual increase in cases of a particular illness might trigger an investigation to determine if there's an outbreak.

Epidemiology is also crucial in **evaluating public health interventions**. For example, when a new vaccine is introduced, epidemiologists assess its effectiveness by comparing disease rates before and after its rollout. This ensures that public health strategies are evidence-based and improve health outcomes efficiently.

History and Evolution of Epidemiology

Epidemiology has its roots in ancient civilizations, where people began to observe patterns in disease outbreaks. Early ideas on the causes of disease were often based on superstition, religion, or environmental factors. Hippocrates, often called the "Father of Medicine," was among the first to challenge supernatural explanations of disease. He suggested that disease might be influenced by the environment and living habits. His observations laid the groundwork for future epidemiological thought, though they lacked scientific rigor.

The **17th century** saw the beginnings of more systematic data collection. During the Great Plague of London in 1665, John Graunt, an English statistician, began analyzing death records. His work, "Natural and Political Observations Made Upon the Bills of Mortality," is considered a foundational text for modern epidemiology. Graunt noted differences in mortality rates based on age, gender, and location, pioneering the use of data to understand disease patterns.

The **18th and 19th centuries** marked significant advancements. In the early 1800s, Edward Jenner developed the smallpox vaccine, one of the first successful disease prevention methods based on the concept of immunity. Meanwhile, epidemiology took a major leap forward with the work of **John Snow** in 1854 during a cholera outbreak in London. Snow's investigation of cholera cases led him to map the affected areas and identify the source of the outbreak: a contaminated water pump. His use of spatial analysis and data to identify the disease's source was revolutionary, marking a shift toward evidence-based epidemiology.

Another major contributor was **Florence Nightingale**, a British nurse who used statistical data during the Crimean War to show that poor sanitation was a major cause of death. Her advocacy for hygiene reform in hospitals helped establish the link between environmental conditions and disease, further shaping epidemiological thinking.

The late **19th century** saw a shift in focus with the rise of germ theory, which proposed that microorganisms caused infectious diseases. This theory, championed by scientists like Louis Pasteur and Robert Koch, transformed epidemiology. Koch's postulates outlined how specific bacteria caused specific diseases, enabling epidemiologists to target interventions more precisely. The focus now was on **identifying pathogens** and **understanding transmission**.

In the **20th century**, epidemiology evolved beyond infectious diseases. The field expanded to chronic diseases like heart disease, cancer, and diabetes, which required different methods to study their longer-term progression. The Framingham Heart Study, launched in 1948, is a prime example of how epidemiology adapted to tackle non-communicable diseases. This study followed a large population over decades to track risk factors for cardiovascular disease, demonstrating the power of longitudinal data in understanding chronic health conditions.

The development of **biostatistics** also was key in the evolution of epidemiology. By incorporating statistical techniques, epidemiologists could better assess associations between risk factors and diseases. This allowed for more precise risk predictions and the ability to control for confounding variables in studies.

The late **20th and early 21st centuries** saw epidemiology embrace new technologies and expand into **molecular and genetic epidemiology**. This approach looks at how genetic factors interact with environmental exposures to influence disease risk. Technologies like genome sequencing and bioinformatics allow researchers to identify genetic predispositions and study their interaction with lifestyle factors.

Additionally, the **HIV/AIDS epidemic** in the 1980s brought new urgency to epidemiology. The rapid global spread of the virus and the need to understand its transmission led to advancements in both **surveillance systems** and **public health interventions**.

Today, epidemiology continues to evolve, incorporating **big data** and **artificial intelligence**. These technologies allow for real-time monitoring of disease

3

outbreaks and more sophisticated modeling of disease trends. For example, during the COVID-19 pandemic, epidemiologists relied on these tools to track the spread of the virus, assess public health interventions, and predict future outbreaks.

Key Roles of an Epidemiologist

Epidemiologists serve as the foundation of public health, using science and data to investigate patterns of disease and health-related events. Their roles span various responsibilities, from data collection and analysis to public health interventions. These professionals work to protect populations from illness, injury, and death by identifying disease causes and developing prevention strategies.

One of the primary roles of an epidemiologist is **disease surveillance**. Surveillance involves the continuous collection, analysis, and interpretation of health data. This helps epidemiologists identify emerging health threats, track disease trends, and detect outbreaks early. For instance, during the COVID-19 pandemic, epidemiologists had a key role in tracking the virus's spread and its variants. Surveillance allows public health agencies to monitor whether diseases are increasing or decreasing and whether interventions are working.

Epidemiologists are also deeply involved in **outbreak investigations**. When a disease spreads unexpectedly, these professionals identify the source and develop strategies to control it. They collect data on who is getting sick, where the cases are concentrated, and how the disease is spreading. By analyzing this information, epidemiologists can determine the **pathways of transmission**. For example, in the case of foodborne illnesses, epidemiologists may trace the outbreak back to a contaminated food product and then recommend recalls or other public health actions to stop further spread.

Another vital role is in **study design and research**. Epidemiologists design studies to investigate the causes of diseases and health conditions. They choose from different study types, such as cohort studies, case-control studies, and randomized controlled trials, depending on the research question. Cohort studies, for example, follow a group of people over time to see who develops a particular condition, while case-control studies compare people with a disease to those without it to identify risk factors. This research forms the backbone of public health knowledge, guiding interventions and policy.

Data analysis is central to the work of epidemiologists. After collecting health data, they use statistical methods to identify patterns and relationships between risk factors and diseases. For example, they might analyze the data from a community to see if air pollution levels correlate with asthma rates. The results of these analyses provide evidence that helps guide public health policies. In modern epidemiology, the use of biostatistics and computer modeling is essential for interpreting complex datasets and making accurate predictions about future health trends.

Epidemiologists are also tasked with **communicating findings** to policymakers, healthcare professionals, and the public. Effective communication is important for translating scientific data into actionable public health recommendations. When presenting their findings, epidemiologists must simplify complex information without losing scientific accuracy. Whether it's advising government agencies during a pandemic or providing information on vaccination programs, clear communication ensures that interventions are both understood and implemented.

In addition to dealing with infectious diseases, many epidemiologists focus on **chronic disease epidemiology**. Chronic diseases such as diabetes, cancer, and heart disease are leading causes of death worldwide. Epidemiologists who specialize in this area study risk factors like diet, exercise, and genetic predispositions. They work to identify patterns in the development of these diseases and propose prevention strategies to reduce incidence rates. For example, the identification of smoking as a major risk factor for lung cancer led to widespread public health campaigns and policies aimed at reducing smoking rates.

Epidemiologists also be important in **evaluating public health interventions**. Once a program, such as a vaccination campaign, is implemented, epidemiologists assess its effectiveness. They analyze whether the intervention has successfully reduced the incidence of disease and make recommendations for improvements. This role is essential for ensuring that resources are used effectively and that public health strategies are evidence-based.

In emergency situations, epidemiologists often act as **field investigators**. They may travel to areas affected by disease outbreaks, natural disasters, or other health emergencies to collect data, provide recommendations, and implement control measures. Their on-the-ground work helps contain disease spread and mitigate health crises. This requires quick decision-making and adaptability, as they must work in unpredictable and often challenging environments.

Epidemiologists' roles, whether in data analysis, outbreak investigation, or public health communication, are essential for protecting population health and preventing disease.

Health and Disease: Basic Concepts

Health is commonly defined as a state of complete physical, mental, and social well-being, not merely the absence of disease or infirmity. This broad definition highlights that health involves more than the physical body—it encompasses mental and emotional states as well. Meanwhile, disease refers to any abnormal condition of the body or mind that causes discomfort, dysfunction, or distress. Disease can be caused by a variety of factors, including pathogens, genetic mutations, environmental exposures, or lifestyle choices.

Understanding health requires an appreciation of the balance between different bodily systems. The body constantly strives to maintain **homeostasis**, a stable internal environment, through processes like temperature regulation and maintaining pH levels in the blood. When a system is disrupted, whether by infection, injury, or chronic stress, homeostasis is affected, potentially leading to disease.

There are two main categories of disease: **infectious and non-infectious**. Infectious diseases are caused by microorganisms such as bacteria, viruses, fungi, or parasites. These diseases can spread from one person to another, either directly (through physical contact, respiratory droplets, or sexual transmission) or indirectly (through contaminated water, food, or surfaces). Examples include tuberculosis, influenza, and COVID-19. Preventing and controlling infectious diseases often involves **public health interventions** like vaccination, sanitation, and quarantine measures.

Non-infectious diseases, on the other hand, are not spread through pathogens but develop due to factors like genetics, lifestyle, or environmental conditions. **Chronic diseases**, such as heart disease, diabetes, and cancer, fall into this category. They often develop over long periods and are influenced by behaviors like smoking, diet, and physical activity. Managing non-infectious diseases typically involves **behavioral changes**, medical treatments, and, in some cases, surgery.

Another key concept in understanding health is **risk factors**. A risk factor is anything that increases a person's chance of developing a disease. Risk factors can be classified as **modifiable** (things you can change) or **non-modifiable** (things you cannot change). Modifiable risk factors include smoking, diet, and exercise habits, while non-modifiable factors include age, gender, and genetic predispositions. Epidemiologists study these risk factors to develop strategies for prevention and treatment.

Health and disease also exist on a **spectrum**. For example, many chronic diseases develop gradually, and the body can move between states of wellness and illness. Conditions like hypertension or early-stage diabetes may not show symptoms but still affect the body's ability to function optimally. Identifying diseases in these early stages can help prevent more serious health problems later on, which is why **screening programs** and **preventive care** are crucial components of modern healthcare.

The **social determinants of health** are another important concept. These include factors like income, education, employment, social support, and the environment in which people live. These elements can profoundly influence health outcomes. For instance, people with lower incomes may have less access to healthcare services, nutritious food, or safe housing, making them more susceptible to diseases. Understanding these social factors is vital for addressing health disparities in different populations.

Public health interventions often focus on **promoting health** rather than just treating disease. Preventive measures like vaccination campaigns, promoting physical activity, and anti-smoking programs aim to reduce the incidence of diseases before they occur. Health promotion encourages individuals to adopt healthier behaviors and empowers communities with the knowledge and resources to protect their health.

In contrast, treating disease involves **diagnosing** and **managing** illness once it's present. This could involve medications, surgeries, or lifestyle modifications depending on the condition. For instance, treating a bacterial infection might require antibiotics, while managing chronic conditions like diabetes would involve continuous monitoring of blood sugar levels, medication, and lifestyle changes.

The concept of **immunity** also is important in the relationship between health and disease. Immunity refers to the body's ability to resist infections, either through natural defenses (like the skin or immune cells) or acquired protection (like vaccination). The **immune system** is the body's defense network against pathogens. When it functions properly, it can destroy harmful invaders before they cause illness. However, when the immune system is weakened or malfunctions, it can lead to increased susceptibility to infections or autoimmune diseases, where the body mistakenly attacks its own cells.

Population vs. Individual Health Perspectives

When we talk about health, there are two main perspectives to consider: **individual health** and **population health**. Each has its own set of goals, challenges, and methods of addressing disease. Understanding the distinction between these two perspectives is important for creating effective healthcare policies and interventions.

The **individual health perspective** focuses on the health and well-being of a single person. This approach is common in clinical settings where healthcare professionals treat individual patients. Physicians diagnose diseases, prescribe treatments, and provide personalized care based on the specific needs of the person. Individual health is often about managing specific conditions—whether acute or chronic—through a tailored treatment plan that considers the person's genetics, environment, lifestyle, and preferences.

In contrast, the **population health perspective** looks at the health outcomes of a group of people, whether defined by geography, occupation, or demographic characteristics. Rather than focusing on individual cases, population health addresses broader health trends within communities or regions. Epidemiologists and public health officials work in this area, identifying patterns and causes of diseases to develop preventive measures that benefit the entire population. For example, they might study obesity rates in a particular city or analyze how air pollution affects respiratory health across different communities.

One of the key differences between these perspectives is the **scale of intervention**. At the individual level, healthcare focuses on treating illness once it's diagnosed, offering specific solutions like medications, surgery, or lifestyle recommendations. Meanwhile, population health emphasizes prevention on a larger scale, such as through public health campaigns, vaccination drives, or sanitation improvements. Population health often addresses the **social determinants of health**, like income, education, and access to healthcare services, aiming to reduce disparities and promote overall well-being.

Another important difference is in how **risk** is managed. Individual health focuses on personal risk factors, such as smoking, diet, or family history of disease. For example, a physician might advise a patient with high cholesterol to adopt a healthier diet and exercise routine to prevent heart disease. In contrast, population health looks at risk on a broader scale, identifying trends that affect entire groups. Public health policies might be designed to reduce these risks through community-wide initiatives—like banning smoking in public places or improving access to nutritious food in low-income neighborhoods.

The **goals** of these perspectives also differ. Individual health aims to improve or maintain the health of a single person, ensuring that they can live a healthy and productive life. Population health aims to improve the health outcomes of entire communities, often focusing on preventing disease before it happens. For example, while a doctor may treat a patient's asthma, a public health official may work to reduce air pollution in a city to prevent asthma cases from increasing.

Data collection is also handled differently. In individual healthcare, medical data is collected through patient histories, lab tests, and clinical observations. This data helps physicians make decisions about diagnosis and treatment. In population health, data is often collected on a much larger scale through surveys, health records, and disease registries. This data is then used to track disease trends, identify at-risk populations, and evaluate the success of public health interventions.

While individual health care is reactive—responding to illnesses as they occur—population health is proactive, aiming to prevent diseases and promote well-being across entire populations. Both perspectives are essential, but they address health in different ways. Together, they contribute to a more comprehensive understanding of health and how to improve it at both the personal and community levels.

The Epidemiologic Triangle: Host, Agent, Environment

The **epidemiologic triangle** is a key model used in epidemiology to explain how diseases develop and spread. It focuses on three critical components: the **host**, the **agent**, and the **environment**. Understanding how these components interact helps epidemiologists identify the causes of diseases and find ways to prevent or control them.

The **host** refers to the organism—usually a human or animal—that can be affected by the disease. In the context of infectious diseases, the host's biological characteristics are critical in determining vulnerability. Factors such as age, genetics, immune status, and lifestyle choices (like diet, exercise, or smoking) can make a host more or less susceptible to disease. For example, older adults or those with weakened immune systems are more likely to develop severe complications from viruses like the flu or COVID-19. **Host factors** also include behaviors that expose individuals to pathogens, such as unprotected sex increasing the risk of sexually transmitted infections.

The **agent** is the cause of the disease. In infectious diseases, this could be a virus, bacterium, fungus, or parasite. Different agents have unique properties that affect how they spread, how they cause illness, and how severe the resulting disease will be. For instance, the influenza virus spreads easily through respiratory droplets, making it a highly contagious agent. In non-infectious diseases, the agent could be a chemical (like lead), radiation, or other environmental exposures (such as allergens that trigger asthma). In the case of chronic diseases, risk factors like high cholesterol or smoking can be considered agents that contribute to conditions like heart disease or lung cancer.

The **environment** includes all external factors that affect the interaction between the host and the agent. These factors can be physical, social, or biological. Physical environments include things like climate, geography, or pollution levels. For instance, areas with high humidity may promote the growth of mold, which can increase respiratory diseases like asthma. Social environments encompass factors like living conditions, socioeconomic status, and access to healthcare. In densely populated urban areas, diseases can spread more rapidly due to close contact between individuals. The biological environment involves the presence of other organisms, like mosquitoes in malaria-endemic regions, which can serve as vectors carrying the disease from one host to another.

The **interaction of host, agent, and environment** determines the likelihood and severity of disease. For example, in the case of malaria, the host could be a human living in a tropical region (environment) where mosquitoes (the agent's vector) thrive. The interaction between these factors—mosquitoes transmitting the Plasmodium parasite to humans—leads to the disease. In other cases, changing one component of the triangle can reduce or eliminate disease transmission. Improving sanitation (environment) or vaccinating individuals (strengthening the host) can break the cycle of transmission for many infectious diseases.

Epidemiologists use the epidemiologic triangle to identify **intervention points**. By understanding which element of the triangle can be modified, public health professionals can reduce disease transmission. For instance, in a flu epidemic, vaccinating hosts or encouraging better hygiene practices can reduce the spread. In non-infectious diseases like lung cancer, reducing exposure to the agent (tobacco smoke) through smoking cessation programs can lower disease incidence.

This simple yet powerful model helps epidemiologists analyze and intervene in health problems by targeting one or more aspects of the triangle. Whether through improving host immunity, controlling the agent, or modifying the environment, the epidemiologic triangle remains central to understanding and managing diseases.

Epidemiology's Role in Public Health Policy

Epidemiology is vital in **shaping public health policy** by providing the scientific evidence needed to address health problems at the population level. By identifying patterns, causes, and risk factors of diseases, epidemiologists inform the development of policies aimed at improving health outcomes and reducing disease burden.

One of the most critical roles epidemiology plays in public health policy is **surveillance**. Surveillance involves the ongoing collection and analysis of health data to monitor disease trends and identify emerging health threats. For example, epidemiological surveillance systems were essential during the COVID-19 pandemic, tracking the spread of the virus and guiding governments on when to implement or relax restrictions. Public health policies often rely on this real-time data to respond swiftly to crises, ensuring timely interventions that prevent widespread illness or death.

Epidemiology is also crucial in **risk assessment**. By identifying risk factors for diseases, such as smoking for lung cancer or sedentary lifestyles for heart disease, epidemiologists provide the foundation for creating policies that target these risks. Risk assessments inform policies like smoking bans in public places, regulations on trans fats, or requirements for vaccinations in schools. These interventions are often designed to reduce exposure to known health risks and improve overall population health.

In the area of **disease prevention**, epidemiological studies provide the evidence necessary to design and implement effective preventive measures. For instance, the relationship between the Human Papillomavirus (HPV) and cervical cancer was established through epidemiological research. This led to the development and widespread adoption of HPV vaccination policies, significantly reducing the incidence of cervical cancer in many countries. Epidemiology helps policymakers determine which prevention strategies will be most effective and cost-efficient in reducing disease rates.

Epidemiologists also contribute to **policy evaluation**, helping to determine whether public health interventions are successful. By comparing health outcomes before and after a policy is implemented, epidemiologists can assess its impact. For instance, after the introduction of seatbelt laws, epidemiologists monitored changes in car accident-related injuries and deaths. The data showed a significant reduction, reinforcing the importance of such policies. This kind of evaluation ensures that public health policies are not only effective but also based on solid scientific evidence.

Resource allocation is another area where epidemiology informs policy decisions. Public health resources, such as funding for healthcare services, vaccination programs, or health education campaigns, are often limited. Epidemiological data helps prioritize which health issues should receive the most attention and funding based on their impact on public health. For example, in areas with high rates of HIV transmission, epidemiological studies can guide the distribution of antiretroviral therapy and preventive measures, ensuring that resources are directed where they will have the greatest impact.

Epidemiology also has a key role in addressing **health disparities**. By analyzing data on how diseases affect different populations, epidemiologists can identify vulnerable groups who are at higher risk due to factors such as socioeconomic status, race, or geography. This information can guide public health policies aimed at reducing disparities. For instance, epidemiological studies highlighting higher rates of diabetes in low-income communities may lead to policies improving access to healthy foods or creating community health programs that focus on diabetes prevention and management.

Global health policies are often shaped by epidemiological research. The World Health Organization (WHO) and other global health bodies rely on epidemiological data to create international guidelines and policies for controlling diseases like malaria, tuberculosis, and HIV/AIDS. Epidemiologists track disease patterns across countries, providing the evidence necessary for coordinated international responses to health crises.

Understanding Disease Distribution: Time, Place, and Person

To understand how diseases spread and affect populations, epidemiologists focus on three critical elements: **time**, **place**, and **person**. These factors help identify patterns in disease distribution, which are essential for diagnosing public health issues, creating prevention strategies, and controlling outbreaks.

The **time** component refers to how the occurrence of disease changes over different periods. This could be short-term, such as hourly or daily variations, or long-term, like seasonal trends or year-to-year patterns. Analyzing the time aspect can reveal important information about the **natural history of a disease**, including when cases are likely to peak and decline. For example, influenza tends to show clear **seasonal patterns**, with higher incidence in the colder months due to factors like increased indoor crowding and the virus thriving in cooler temperatures. By recognizing these patterns, public health officials can better plan vaccination campaigns and allocate resources during peak times.

Epidemiologists also track **epidemic curves**, which display the number of new cases over time. These curves can help distinguish between different types of outbreaks. For instance, a **point-source outbreak**, like food poisoning from a contaminated meal, will show a sharp rise and fall in cases within a short period. In contrast, a **propagated outbreak**, where disease spreads from person to person (as in measles or COVID-19), will have a more gradual rise and fall, as the disease spreads through the population. Recognizing these patterns can help epidemiologists determine the source and transmission method of the disease.

The **place** element refers to the geographical distribution of diseases. This helps identify where diseases are more prevalent, whether within a specific neighborhood, city, country, or region. Geographical data can highlight **clusters** of diseases, suggesting localized outbreaks or environmental risk factors. For instance, diseases like malaria are highly concentrated in tropical regions because the Anopheles mosquito, the disease vector, thrives in those climates. Similarly, the distribution of diseases like lung cancer might show higher rates in industrial areas with high pollution levels.

Mapping diseases geographically through tools like **geographic information systems (GIS)** allows epidemiologists to visualize where disease cases are occurring and how they spread. For example, during the Ebola outbreak in West Africa, maps of disease cases helped health officials target affected regions with medical aid and quarantine measures. Such mapping also helps in the containment of diseases by identifying potential "hot spots" where interventions can be deployed more efficiently.

Finally, the **person** factor looks at the individual characteristics that influence who gets sick. These characteristics include **demographics** like age, gender, and race, as well as **behaviors** such as smoking, diet, or occupation. Understanding the person factor is essential for identifying which groups are at higher risk for certain diseases. For instance, older adults are more likely to experience severe complications from diseases like COVID-19 or the flu, while children are more susceptible to infections like chickenpox or measles.

Epidemiologists also examine **social factors**, such as socioeconomic status or access to healthcare, which can greatly influence disease distribution. People with limited access to healthcare might experience delayed diagnoses or inadequate treatment, leading to higher morbidity and mortality rates. This was seen in the HIV/AIDS epidemic, where marginalized populations without access to preventive measures like testing and antiretroviral therapy were disproportionately affected.

In addition to demographic factors, **genetic predispositions** have a role in how diseases affect individuals. For example, certain cancers, such as breast cancer, can be more common in people with specific genetic mutations (e.g., BRCA1 or BRCA2). Knowing this allows for targeted screening and prevention efforts in at-risk populations.

By analyzing disease distribution in terms of time, place, and person, epidemiologists can uncover critical information about how diseases spread, who is most at risk, and what factors contribute to outbreaks. This understanding is essential for developing effective public health interventions, from vaccination programs to disease containment strategies. Each of these elements helps to form a comprehensive picture of disease dynamics, providing the evidence necessary for informed public health decisions.

Key Metrics: Morbidity, Mortality, and Risk

Epidemiologists use several key metrics to understand disease patterns and inform public health strategies. Among the most important are **morbidity**, **mortality**, and **risk**. Each of these metrics provides valuable insight into the impact of diseases on populations and helps guide decision-making in healthcare and policy.

Morbidity refers to the presence of illness or disease within a population. It encompasses both the incidence (new cases) and prevalence (total cases) of diseases. **Incidence** measures how many new cases of a disease occur during a specific time frame, typically expressed as a rate per 1,000 or 100,000 people. For example, if a city of 100,000 people records 500 new cases of influenza in a month, the incidence rate is 500 per 100,000. This metric helps epidemiologists assess the spread of acute diseases like infectious outbreaks.

Prevalence, on the other hand, indicates the total number of people living with a particular disease at a given time, regardless of when the disease was first diagnosed. It is particularly useful for understanding the burden of **chronic diseases**. For example, the prevalence of diabetes in a population tells us how widespread the condition is, which helps in allocating healthcare resources, developing prevention programs, and planning for long-term care needs. **High prevalence** indicates a significant public health issue that requires sustained attention, even if the disease is not rapidly spreading.

Mortality refers to the number of deaths caused by a disease within a population. The **mortality rate** is typically expressed as deaths per 1,000 or 100,000 people over a certain period, such as a year. Mortality data provides insight into the **severity of a disease** and its impact on public health. For example, diseases like Ebola have a high mortality rate, meaning a significant proportion of those who become infected die, which signals an urgent need for rapid containment and treatment efforts. In contrast, diseases with low mortality rates, such as the common cold, may cause widespread illness but are less deadly.

Epidemiologists also examine **cause-specific mortality**, which breaks down deaths by specific causes, such as cancer or heart disease. This information helps public health officials target interventions more effectively. For instance, if heart disease is responsible for a high percentage of deaths in a population, policymakers might prioritize initiatives to reduce risk factors like smoking, poor diet, and physical inactivity.

Risk is a central concept in epidemiology that refers to the **likelihood** of an individual or group developing a disease. **Risk factors** are characteristics or behaviors that increase this likelihood, such as smoking for lung cancer or high blood pressure for stroke. Epidemiologists use measures like **relative risk** and **odds ratios** to quantify the strength of the association between risk factors and disease outcomes.

For example, if a study finds that smokers are 10 times more likely to develop lung cancer than non-smokers, the relative risk is 10. This means that smoking is a significant risk factor for lung cancer. Understanding risk allows healthcare providers and public health officials to identify individuals or groups at high risk and implement **preventive measures**, such as smoking cessation programs or regular screenings for at-risk populations.

Epidemiologists also differentiate between **absolute risk** and **relative risk**. **Absolute risk** refers to the actual chance of developing a disease over a certain period, while **relative risk** compares the risk between different groups. Both are important for communicating risk to the public and making informed decisions about prevention and treatment strategies.

How Epidemiology Informs Public Health Interventions

Epidemiology provides the foundational data and analysis that inform **public health interventions**. By systematically studying the patterns, causes, and effects of health and disease conditions in populations, epidemiologists help identify health problems, evaluate risks, and design strategies to prevent or control diseases. Public health interventions are largely based on the evidence provided by epidemiological research, allowing for more effective targeting of resources and programs.

One of the key ways epidemiology informs interventions is through **disease surveillance**. Surveillance involves the continuous collection, analysis, and interpretation of health data, which is critical for detecting emerging health threats and monitoring trends over time. When an outbreak occurs, like during the COVID-19 pandemic, real-time surveillance allows public health officials to track the spread of the disease and develop interventions such as quarantine measures, social distancing, and vaccination campaigns. By understanding when and where diseases are spreading, epidemiologists guide public health decisions to limit further transmission and protect vulnerable populations.

Epidemiological research also identifies **risk factors** for diseases, which in turn shapes preventive interventions. For example, studies have long demonstrated that smoking is a significant risk factor for lung cancer and cardiovascular diseases. As a result, many countries have implemented **anti-smoking policies**, such as cigarette taxes, smoking bans in public places, and public awareness campaigns about the dangers of smoking. Similarly, epidemiological studies linking poor diet and physical inactivity to obesity and diabetes have led to **health promotion interventions** that encourage healthier eating habits and increased physical activity. By pinpointing modifiable risk factors, epidemiologists provide the evidence needed to reduce exposure to those risks through public health programs.

Epidemiology also informs the development and implementation of **vaccination programs**. The relationship between epidemiology and vaccines is well established, with epidemiological studies determining which populations are most at risk and which diseases are preventable through vaccination. For example, global efforts to eradicate diseases like polio have relied heavily on epidemiological data to track where cases are occurring, identify gaps in vaccine coverage, and target areas for intensified vaccination efforts. Epidemiology also helps guide decisions about **booster doses**, as seen in the context of the COVID-19 vaccine, where studies on immunity duration informed policies on additional doses.

In the case of **chronic diseases**, epidemiology is important in shaping long-term public health strategies. For instance, epidemiological studies on heart disease have identified key risk factors, including high cholesterol, high blood pressure, smoking, and lack of physical activity. This research has led to widespread public health campaigns promoting heart health, encouraging regular exercise, healthier diets, and smoking cessation. In many countries, public health interventions such as **blood pressure screening programs**, **cholesterol checks**, and **public awareness campaigns** around healthy lifestyle choices are based on this epidemiological data.

Epidemiology also provides essential data for **resource allocation** in public health. Health systems often have limited resources, and epidemiologists help prioritize how those resources are used by identifying where disease burden is highest. For example, if epidemiological data shows a high incidence of malaria in specific regions, public health officials can target those areas with **insecticide-treated bed nets**, **antimalarial medications**, and **mosquito control programs**. In the case of emerging infectious diseases, such as Ebola outbreaks, epidemiological data helps determine where to deploy medical teams, supplies, and resources to contain the disease effectively.

One of the key aspects of epidemiology is its ability to inform **evaluation of public health interventions**. After a program is implemented, epidemiologists track its impact on disease rates and overall health outcomes. For example, following the introduction of HPV vaccines, epidemiologists have monitored the decline in cervical cancer cases, providing evidence that the vaccination program is working. This process of **program evaluation** is critical for ensuring that public health interventions are effective and for making necessary adjustments if the desired outcomes are not being achieved.

Epidemiology also is key in managing **non-communicable diseases** (NCDs), which are responsible for a significant portion of global mortality. Studies on NCDs, such as diabetes, heart disease, and cancer, have provided the evidence needed to implement preventive interventions like promoting **healthy eating**, **physical activity**, and **early screening programs**. Epidemiological data has also informed the creation of public policies, such as **food labeling regulations** and **restrictions on the marketing of unhealthy products**, which aim to reduce the burden of NCDs on populations.

In public health emergencies, **field epidemiology** becomes particularly important. Epidemiologists often conduct rapid investigations to identify the source and spread of diseases during outbreaks. For example, in the case of foodborne illnesses, field epidemiologists might trace the outbreak to a specific contaminated food product and work with public health authorities to recall the product, thereby preventing further illness. This investigative role is crucial for implementing **quick, targeted interventions** that can stop the spread of disease.

Epidemiology also supports **policy development** by providing the data needed to make informed decisions about public health laws and regulations. For instance, epidemiological studies on traffic-related injuries have led to the introduction of **seatbelt laws** and **drunk driving regulations**. Similarly, studies on air pollution and respiratory diseases have contributed to **environmental regulations** that aim to reduce harmful emissions and improve air quality.

CHAPTER 2: MEASURES OF DISEASE FREQUENCY

Incidence and Prevalence

In epidemiology, two key measures used to understand how disease affects populations are **incidence** and **prevalence**. Both provide insights, but they focus on different aspects of disease frequency. Knowing the distinction between them is critical for analyzing and responding to public health issues effectively.

Incidence refers to the number of **new cases** of a disease that occur in a specific population during a defined period. It focuses on the **rate of disease development**. This measure is particularly useful for understanding how quickly a disease is spreading and for identifying emerging health threats. To calculate incidence, epidemiologists need two pieces of data: the number of new cases and the population at risk during a specified time period.

For example, if you are tracking influenza cases in a city with 100,000 people over a one-year period, and 1,000 new cases are reported, the incidence rate would be 1,000 per 100,000 people per year. Incidence is expressed as a rate, often per 1,000 or 100,000 people, to standardize comparisons across different populations or timeframes.

There are two types of incidence measurements: **cumulative incidence** and **incidence rate** (or incidence density). **Cumulative incidence** is the proportion of individuals who develop the disease over a specific period. It is simple to understand and calculate when you know the exact number of people at risk at the start of the period. For instance, if 500 out of 10,000 people develop a disease over a year, the cumulative incidence would be 500 divided by 10,000, or 0.05 (5%).

The **incidence rate**, on the other hand, takes into account the time each individual in the population is at risk. It is a more precise measure when people enter and leave the population or are at risk for different lengths of time. The incidence rate is expressed as the number of new cases per person-time at risk. If 1,000 new cases occur over 50,000 person-years, the incidence rate would be 20 cases per 1,000 person-years.

In contrast, **prevalence** is the total number of **existing cases** of a disease in a population at a specific point in time or over a defined period. Prevalence tells us how widespread a disease is, rather than how quickly it is developing. It includes both **new and ongoing cases**, making it particularly useful for chronic conditions like diabetes or hypertension, where the goal is to manage the total burden of disease.

Prevalence is calculated as the number of people with the disease divided by the total population, expressed as a proportion or percentage. For example, if 2,000 people in a population of 100,000 have diabetes, the prevalence would be 2,000 divided by 100,000, or 0.02, which means a 2% prevalence rate.

There are two types of prevalence: **point prevalence** and **period prevalence**. **Point prevalence** refers to the proportion of people with a disease at a specific moment in time. For instance, if a survey conducted on January 1st shows that 1% of the population has a particular condition, that is the point prevalence. **Period prevalence** measures the proportion of people with a disease over a defined period, such as a year. It accounts for all cases present at any point during the time period, including those who developed the disease before the period began.

Incidence and prevalence measure different aspects of disease frequency. Incidence focuses on the occurrence of new cases and is useful for studying the causes and risk factors of diseases. It helps public health officials identify outbreaks or trends in emerging diseases. Prevalence, on the other hand, captures the overall burden of disease in a population and is key for planning healthcare services, allocating resources, and understanding the long-term impact of chronic conditions.

It's important to remember that while incidence reflects the **risk** of getting the disease, prevalence reflects the **total burden** of the disease within the population. For chronic diseases, where individuals may live with the condition for years, prevalence can remain high even if the incidence is relatively low. This is why **both measures are important** for understanding the full picture of disease dynamics in a population.

Person-Time Measures

In epidemiology, **person-time** is a way to account for both the number of individuals in a study and the amount of time each individual is observed, particularly in studies where follow-up periods differ among participants. It's a critical concept for understanding how disease incidence is measured in dynamic populations, where not everyone is at risk for the same amount of time.

Person-time measures the **sum of the time** that each individual in a population is at risk of developing a particular disease. It's typically expressed as **person-years**, though it can also be represented as person-months or person-days depending on the study duration. For example, if 100 people are followed for one year, the study would accumulate 100 person-years of observation. If 10 people are followed for 5 years, that also adds up to 50 person-years.

This method is especially useful in cohort studies, where participants may enter or exit the study at different times, or where they may die, move away, or otherwise stop being at risk. **Person-time compensates for these variations**, providing a more accurate measure of the disease rate in a population over time.

The **incidence rate** is often calculated using person-time as the denominator. For example, if a study follows 1,000 people for a total of 10,000 person-years and 50 people develop a disease, the incidence rate would be 50 cases per 10,000 person-years. This can be converted to a more interpretable figure by dividing the result, giving 5 cases per 1,000 person-years. Person-time allows epidemiologists to account for varying follow-up times, which is essential for studies with long follow-up periods or large populations.

Person-time also accommodates **censored data**. Censoring occurs when participants are lost to follow-up, withdraw from the study, or when the study ends before they develop the disease. In these cases, their person-time is still counted up to the point of their last known observation, giving a more complete view of the total time the population was at risk.

By using person-time measures, epidemiologists can calculate disease rates that are more reflective of the actual risk within the population. This is especially important for studies involving chronic diseases, where the risk of disease may increase over long periods, and not all participants remain at risk for the entire study duration.

Standardized Rates and Ratios

Standardized rates and **ratios** are used to make fair comparisons of disease frequencies between populations with different structures, particularly when those populations vary by age, gender, or other demographic factors. These measures adjust for these differences, allowing epidemiologists to compare health outcomes more accurately.

A **crude rate** is simply the total number of cases of a disease in a population divided by the total population. However, crude rates can be misleading when comparing populations that differ significantly in their demographic makeup. For example, if you were comparing heart disease rates between two populations, one with a much older population and one with a younger demographic, the crude rate in the older population would likely be higher simply because heart disease is more common in older adults. To correct for these differences, epidemiologists use **age-standardized rates** (also called age-adjusted rates).

Standardization can be done using **direct** or **indirect methods**. The **direct method** involves applying the age-specific rates of the study population to a standard population structure. This standard population could be the total population of a country or a global reference population. For example, if you want to compare cancer rates between two countries with different age distributions, you would apply the age-specific cancer rates from each country to a single standard population structure. This adjustment removes the effect of the differing age distributions, allowing a more accurate comparison of cancer risk.

In contrast, the **indirect method** is often used when age-specific rates for the study population are unknown or unreliable. In this case, the age-specific rates from the standard population are applied to the age distribution of the study population. This results in the calculation of an **expected number of cases**, which can then be compared to the observed number of cases in the study population. The **standardized mortality ratio (SMR)** or **standardized incidence ratio (SIR)** is a common outcome of the indirect method. These ratios compare the observed number of deaths (or disease cases) to the number expected if the study population had the same age-specific rates as the standard population.

The **SMR** or **SIR** is calculated as:

$$SMR = (Observed\ cases\ /\ Expected\ cases) \times 100$$

For example, if a mining community has an SMR of 150 for lung cancer, this indicates that the lung cancer rate in that population is 50% higher than what would be expected based on the standard population's rates. Ratios above 100 indicate a higher-than-expected rate, while ratios below 100 indicate a lower-than-expected rate.

Standardized rates and ratios are crucial in **epidemiological comparisons** because they ensure that observed differences in disease frequency aren't simply due to variations in population structure. These adjustments allow public health officials to identify true differences in disease risk and to develop interventions that target the actual causes of those differences, rather than being misled by demographic factors.

Adjusting for Age and Other Demographic Factors

When studying disease frequency, adjusting for **age** and other demographic factors is essential to obtain accurate and meaningful comparisons between populations. Diseases often affect specific age groups differently, and failing to account for these differences can lead to misleading conclusions. Adjusting for demographic factors ensures that comparisons between different populations or over time reflect true differences in disease risk, rather than differences in the underlying population structure.

Age is one of the most significant demographic factors in epidemiology because many diseases are more common in certain age groups. For example, heart disease and cancer are more prevalent in older adults, while conditions like asthma or certain infections are more common in children. If you compare the crude rate of heart disease between a population with a large number of older people and one with mostly younger individuals, the rate in the older population will naturally appear higher due to age, even if the actual risk of heart disease at each age is similar in both groups. This is where **age adjustment** becomes critical.

There are two primary methods for adjusting for age: **direct standardization** and **indirect standardization**. Each method helps to account for age distribution differences, though they are used in different contexts depending on the available data.

Direct standardization involves applying age-specific rates from the study population to a standard population with a fixed age structure. This method is most useful when you have reliable age-specific disease rates for each population you're comparing. Let's say you are comparing lung cancer rates between two countries. If one country has a much older population than the other, its crude lung cancer rate may be higher simply due to age. By applying the age-specific rates from each country to a standard population (such as the overall world population or a national reference population), you can adjust for these differences. The resulting **age-adjusted rate** reflects what the lung cancer rate would be if both countries had the same age distribution, making the comparison fairer and more meaningful.

For example, if the crude lung cancer rate is 50 per 100,000 people in one country and 80 per 100,000 in another, age adjustment might reveal that, when controlling for age, the adjusted rates are actually closer, say 55 per 100,000 versus 60 per 100,000. This adjustment shows that the apparent difference in crude rates was largely due to the older population in the second country, not a greater underlying risk of lung cancer.

Indirect standardization, on the other hand, is used when age-specific rates for the study population are unavailable or unreliable. In this method, you apply the age-specific rates from a standard population to the age structure of your study population. This gives an **expected number of cases**, which can then be compared to the **observed number of cases** in the study population. The result is typically expressed as a **standardized mortality ratio (SMR)** or **standardized incidence ratio (SIR)**, which indicates whether the disease or mortality rate in the study population is higher or lower than expected based on the standard population's rates.

The **SMR** is particularly useful for studying occupational groups or small populations where disease cases may be too few for reliable age-specific rates. For instance, if a mining community has an SMR of 120 for lung cancer, this indicates that the lung cancer rate in the community is 20% higher than expected based on the rates in the general population. This method adjusts for differences in age distribution but doesn't provide an actual rate like direct standardization does; instead, it provides a ratio comparing observed to expected cases.

In addition to age, other **demographic factors** such as **gender, race**, and **socioeconomic status** often influence disease distribution and must be adjusted for when comparing populations. For example, certain diseases like breast cancer predominantly affect women, while prostate cancer is specific to men. Gender-specific rates are important to avoid skewing results when populations differ significantly in their gender makeup. Similarly, racial and ethnic groups may experience different disease risks due to genetic, environmental, or cultural factors. Adjusting for race and ethnicity is critical when studying conditions like hypertension or diabetes, which may have higher prevalence in certain racial groups.

Socioeconomic status (SES) is another key demographic factor that impacts disease frequency. People with lower SES often face higher rates of certain diseases due to limited access to healthcare, poorer living conditions, and greater exposure to risk factors like smoking or unhealthy diets. Adjusting for SES can help isolate the effects of these factors from the true underlying risk of disease. For instance, comparing disease rates between high-income and low-income neighborhoods without adjusting for SES could exaggerate the impact of disease in poorer areas without accounting for the broader social determinants of health.

Adjusting for demographic factors like age, gender, race, and SES is fundamental to measuring disease frequency accurately. These adjustments allow epidemiologists to disentangle the effects of population structure from the true risks of disease, ensuring that public health policies and interventions are based on reliable data.

CHAPTER 3: STUDY DESIGNS IN EPIDEMIOLOGY

Observational vs. Experimental Studies

In epidemiology, **study designs** are essential for investigating health issues and understanding disease patterns. Two main categories of study designs are **observational studies** and **experimental studies**. Each approach has its own strengths, limitations, and applications, depending on the type of health problem being studied.

Observational studies focus on watching and recording what naturally happens in a population without manipulating any variables. In these studies, researchers collect data on exposures and outcomes as they occur, but they do not intervene. Observational studies are valuable for identifying associations between risk factors and diseases and are often used when experimental studies are not feasible or ethical. For instance, you can't ethically assign people to smoke cigarettes to study lung cancer development. Instead, you would observe people who already smoke and those who don't, then compare their health outcomes.

There are several types of observational studies, each with distinct features. **Cohort studies** follow groups of people over time, typically starting with individuals who are free of disease. Participants are categorized based on their exposure to certain risk factors, and the researchers track who develops the disease. For example, a cohort study might follow a group of smokers and non-smokers over several years to see which group is more likely to develop lung cancer. Cohort studies can be **prospective**, meaning the data collection starts before the outcome occurs, or **retrospective**, meaning the study looks back at data that has already been collected. Prospective cohort studies tend to be more reliable, but they require more time and resources.

Another type of observational study is the **case-control study**. In this design, researchers select individuals with the disease (cases) and compare them to individuals without the disease (controls). The goal is to look back in time to determine which risk factors were more common in the cases. Case-control studies are efficient for studying rare diseases or conditions with long latency periods, like certain cancers. However, they rely heavily on participants' memories of past exposures, which can introduce **recall bias**. If cases remember their exposures differently than controls, it could skew the results.

Cross-sectional studies are another observational design. These studies examine a population at a single point in time, measuring both exposure and outcome simultaneously. They are useful for assessing **prevalence**, or how widespread a disease is at a particular moment. For example, a cross-sectional study could assess how many people currently have high blood pressure and how many of those individuals are physically inactive. The limitation of cross-sectional studies is that they cannot determine causality—whether the exposure led to the outcome—since both are measured at the same time.

In contrast to observational studies, **experimental studies** involve **intervention**. In these studies, researchers actively manipulate one or more variables to test a hypothesis. The most common type of experimental study in epidemiology is the **randomized controlled trial (RCT)**. In an RCT, participants are randomly assigned to either an intervention group (which receives the treatment or exposure) or a control group (which does not). This randomization helps reduce **confounding variables**, making RCTs one of the strongest study designs for determining cause-and-effect relationships.

For example, in a study testing a new vaccine, one group of participants would receive the vaccine, while the other group might receive a placebo. Researchers would then compare the outcomes between the two groups to see if the vaccine reduced disease incidence. By randomly assigning participants to different groups, RCTs minimize bias and allow for more reliable conclusions. However, RCTs are often expensive and time-consuming to conduct. They can also raise ethical issues, especially if withholding treatment from a control group could cause harm.

Quasi-experimental studies are similar to RCTs but lack random assignment. In these studies, researchers still intervene by offering a treatment or exposure, but participants aren't randomly assigned to groups. Quasi-experimental designs are used when randomization isn't possible due to logistical or ethical reasons. Though not as strong as RCTs in eliminating bias, these studies still provide useful information about the effects of an intervention.

Cross-Sectional Studies

Cross-sectional studies are a type of observational study that examines a population at a single point in time or over a short period. In these studies, researchers collect data on both exposures (such as risk factors) and outcomes (such as disease presence) simultaneously. Cross-sectional studies are valuable for assessing the **prevalence** of diseases or health conditions and identifying potential associations between exposures and outcomes. However, because both exposure and outcome are measured at the same time, cross-sectional studies cannot determine causality—whether an exposure leads to a particular health outcome.

One of the main uses of cross-sectional studies is in public health for **prevalence estimation**. Prevalence refers to the total number of cases of a disease or condition in a given population at a specific point in time. For example, a cross-sectional study might be used to estimate how many people in a city have high blood pressure at the time of the survey. This type of information is critical for public health planning because it shows the **burden of disease** in a population and helps guide decisions about resource allocation, screening programs, and interventions.

Cross-sectional studies are often conducted using **surveys** or **questionnaires**. Researchers may ask participants about their health status, lifestyle factors (such as smoking or physical activity), and demographic information (such as age, gender, and income). In some cases, cross-sectional studies may also involve **biological measurements**, such as blood tests or physical exams, to collect more objective data on health outcomes. Because they collect data from many people at once, cross-sectional studies are relatively quick and cost-effective compared to other study designs.

Despite these advantages, cross-sectional studies have some important limitations. The most significant is their inability to establish **temporal relationships**—the order in which exposure and outcome occur. For example, if a cross-sectional study finds that people with higher levels of stress have more cases of heart disease, it is impossible to tell whether the stress led to the heart disease or whether having heart disease caused the stress. Without knowing which came first, it is difficult to draw conclusions about cause and effect.

Another limitation is the potential for **selection bias**. Because cross-sectional studies rely on the people who are available and willing to participate at the time of the study, the sample may not be representative of the broader population. For instance, if only healthier individuals are more likely to respond to a health survey, the study could underestimate the true prevalence of a disease. Similarly, people with certain conditions may be more motivated to participate in studies, leading to **overestimation** of disease prevalence.

Despite these drawbacks, cross-sectional studies are widely used in **public health surveillance** to monitor trends in disease prevalence and health behaviors. For example, large national health surveys like the **Behavioral Risk Factor Surveillance System (BRFSS)** in the United States rely on cross-sectional methods to gather data on health behaviors and conditions such as smoking, obesity, and diabetes. These data help identify **high-risk populations** and guide public health interventions.

Cross-sectional studies are also useful for generating **hypotheses** about potential risk factors for diseases. While they cannot prove causality, they can highlight associations that warrant further investigation. For example, if a cross-sectional study finds that people who drink sugary beverages have higher rates of obesity, this could lead to more in-depth research, such as a cohort study or randomized trial, to explore whether sugary beverages cause weight gain.

In some cases, cross-sectional studies can be combined with other study designs to strengthen their findings. For instance, repeated cross-sectional studies—conducted over time but with different participants each time—can provide insights into trends in disease prevalence and risk factors. While each study captures a snapshot of the population at one point in time, analyzing multiple snapshots over time can help identify changes in health patterns and the effectiveness of public health interventions.

Cohort Studies

Cohort studies are a fundamental observational study design in epidemiology, where researchers follow a group of people (a cohort) over time to examine the relationship between exposures and the development of disease. Unlike cross-sectional studies, which capture a snapshot of a population at one point in time, cohort studies follow participants over a longer period, allowing researchers to track changes and see how different exposures affect health outcomes.

In a cohort study, participants are typically classified based on their exposure status at the beginning of the study. For example, in a study looking at the effects of smoking on lung cancer, researchers might group participants into smokers and non-smokers. These groups are then followed over time to observe who develops lung cancer and who doesn't. The **incidence** of disease—the number of new cases over time—is compared between the exposed and unexposed groups, providing insight into whether the exposure is associated with a higher or lower risk of disease.

Cohort studies can be either **prospective** or **retrospective**. In a **prospective cohort study**, researchers recruit participants at the start of the study and follow them forward in time. This allows for a more controlled and accurate collection of exposure data since researchers can directly monitor the participants from the beginning. For example, in the **Framingham Heart Study**, which began in 1948, participants were followed for decades to assess risk factors for cardiovascular disease. Prospective cohort studies are ideal for studying risk factors that may take years or decades to lead to disease, but they require long follow-up periods and significant resources.

In a **retrospective cohort study**, the research begins after both the exposure and the outcome have already occurred. Researchers use existing data—such as medical records or employment histories—to track participants back in time and assess how past exposures influenced disease development. While retrospective cohort studies are quicker and less expensive than prospective studies, they often rely on less accurate or incomplete data, which can limit their reliability.

One of the major strengths of cohort studies is their ability to establish **temporal relationships**—the sequence of events in which the exposure precedes the outcome. This makes cohort studies particularly useful for investigating potential causes of diseases. For example, if a prospective cohort study shows that people who are obese at the start of the study are more likely to develop diabetes over the following decade, this provides strong evidence that obesity is a risk factor for diabetes. The ability to observe the **natural progression** of health conditions over time gives cohort studies a clear advantage in identifying causality compared to cross-sectional studies.

Another strength of cohort studies is their ability to study **multiple outcomes** from a single exposure. For instance, a cohort of smokers can be followed to study not only lung cancer but also other outcomes like heart disease, respiratory conditions, and mortality. This flexibility makes cohort studies a strong framework in epidemiology.

However, cohort studies also have limitations. **Loss to follow-up** is a significant concern, especially in long-term prospective studies. Participants may drop out, move away, or otherwise become unavailable for follow-up, which can introduce bias if those lost to follow-up are systematically different from those who remain. For example, if people with more severe illness are more likely to drop out, the remaining cohort may appear healthier than it actually is.

Another challenge is the potential for **confounding variables**—factors that are associated with both the exposure and the outcome but are not part of the study. For example, in a study of the relationship between exercise and heart disease, age might be a confounder, since older people may exercise less and are also more likely to develop heart disease. To address this, researchers can use statistical techniques to control for confounding factors, but these methods cannot completely eliminate the problem.

Cohort studies are also **resource-intensive**. Prospective studies require long follow-up periods, sometimes spanning decades, and demand significant funding and logistical support to maintain data collection and participant engagement over time. This makes cohort studies less feasible for diseases with long latency periods or for conditions that develop infrequently in the population.

Despite these challenges, cohort studies remain one of the most reliable and informative study designs in epidemiology. Their ability to track disease development over time, establish temporal relationships, and investigate multiple outcomes makes them essential for identifying risk factors and understanding the natural history of diseases.

Case-Control Studies

Case-control studies are a type of observational study used in epidemiology to investigate the causes of diseases, especially rare conditions or those with long latency periods. These studies are **retrospective**, meaning they start with the outcome (disease or condition) and look back in time to identify exposures that may have contributed to that outcome. Case-control studies are particularly efficient when studying diseases that take a long time to develop, such as certain cancers or heart diseases, because they allow researchers to work backward from the disease to possible causes.

In a case-control study, researchers identify two groups of participants: **cases**, who have the disease or condition of interest, and **controls**, who do not have the disease. The key task in case-control studies is to compare the prior exposure to risk factors between the two groups. For example, in a study of lung cancer, cases would be individuals with lung cancer, and controls would be people without lung cancer. Both groups would be questioned about their smoking habits or other relevant exposures in the past. The goal is to determine whether the cases had a higher rate of exposure to the suspected risk factor (like smoking) than the controls.

A major strength of case-control studies is their **efficiency**, especially when studying rare diseases. For conditions like mesothelioma, which has a low incidence rate, it would be impractical to follow a large group of people for many years in a cohort study to wait and see who develops the disease. Instead, case-control studies allow researchers to start with people who already have the disease and look backward to find patterns in exposures. This saves both time and resources.

Another advantage is that **multiple exposures** can be investigated in a single study. Case-control studies can explore different risk factors that may be linked to the disease, such as environmental factors, lifestyle choices, or genetic predispositions. For example, in studying lung cancer, researchers could look at smoking, occupational exposures, air pollution, and genetic factors, all within the same study.

Despite their advantages, case-control studies have significant limitations. One of the primary concerns is **recall bias**. Since the study relies on participants' memories of past exposures, cases may remember their experiences differently from controls. For example, people with lung cancer may more vividly recall smoking habits or environmental exposures, while controls may not remember these details as clearly. This difference in memory can skew the results and make it appear that certain exposures are more strongly linked to the disease than they actually are.

Another limitation is **selection bias**. Choosing appropriate controls is crucial for the validity of a case-control study. Controls should come from the same population as the cases and should be similar to them in key aspects, except for the disease status. If controls are not well-matched to the cases, the comparison may be flawed. For instance, if a study on lung cancer cases selects controls from a hospital where people are receiving treatment for other smoking-related diseases, the controls might be more likely to smoke than the general population, leading to biased results.

Confounding is another challenge in case-control studies. A confounder is a factor that is associated with both the disease and the exposure but is not part of the causal pathway. For example, in a case-control study of heart disease, age could be a confounder if older people are both more likely to have heart disease and more likely to have certain exposures, like less physical activity. Researchers use statistical techniques, such as **multivariate analysis**, to control for confounders, but confounding can never be fully eliminated.

A common measure used in case-control studies is the **odds ratio (OR)**. The odds ratio compares the odds of exposure in the cases to the odds of exposure in the controls. If the odds ratio is greater than 1, this suggests that the exposure is more common among cases and may be associated with an increased risk of disease. For example, an odds ratio of 2 would mean that cases are twice as likely to have been exposed to a risk factor compared to controls.

Nested Case-Control and Case-Cohort Studies

Nested case-control studies and **case-cohort studies** are advanced variations of traditional cohort studies, designed to make use of large cohort data while preserving some of the efficiency seen in case-control studies. These study designs are particularly useful when researchers need to investigate risk factors within an established cohort without having to analyze data for the entire cohort, saving both time and resources.

In a **nested case-control study**, cases and controls are drawn from a cohort that has already been established and followed over time. The cases are individuals within the cohort who develop the disease or outcome of interest, while the controls are selected from those in the same cohort who have not developed the disease by the time the cases occur. For example, in a large cohort study on heart disease, researchers could select individuals who developed heart disease (cases) and compare them to a random sample of those who did not (controls), using data collected from the entire cohort.

One advantage of nested case-control studies is that the **exposure data** has often been collected **prospectively**, meaning it was recorded before the disease developed. This reduces **recall bias**, a common problem in traditional case-control studies. Since all participants are drawn from the same cohort, their exposures were measured at the same time and under the same conditions, providing more accurate and reliable data on risk factors.

Another strength of the nested case-control design is **efficiency**. By selecting only a subset of the cohort for further analysis (the cases and controls), researchers avoid the need to perform costly and time-consuming analyses on the entire cohort. This is particularly useful when the disease is rare or when the cohort is very large, and analyzing every member of the cohort would be impractical.

A limitation of nested case-control studies is that the controls are sampled from individuals who have not yet developed the disease, meaning that if the follow-up continues, some of the controls might eventually become cases. This introduces a slight complication in data analysis, but this can be accounted for with proper statistical adjustments.

Case-cohort studies are similar to nested case-control studies, but they differ in how controls are selected. In a case-cohort study, a **sub-cohort** is randomly selected from the entire original cohort, and this sub-cohort serves as the comparison group for all cases, regardless of when the cases develop. The sub-cohort is established at the beginning of the study and remains constant throughout the follow-up period. All cases that develop in the full cohort, not just in the sub-cohort, are included in the analysis.

This design allows for **multiple outcomes** to be studied simultaneously. Since the sub-cohort represents the larger cohort, it can be used as a control group for different diseases or outcomes that might develop in the cohort. For example, in a study on cardiovascular risk, the same sub-cohort could be used as the control group for cases of heart disease, stroke, and diabetes, reducing the need to repeatedly select new controls for each outcome.

A key benefit of case-cohort studies is that, like nested case-control studies, they allow researchers to analyze exposures prospectively. The exposure data is collected before the outcome develops, which minimizes bias and ensures that the temporal relationship between exposure and outcome is clear. Additionally, the case-cohort design allows for the use of the same control group for multiple outcomes, making it highly **cost-effective** for large cohort studies investigating various diseases.

However, case-cohort studies also have their challenges. Since the sub-cohort is used for multiple comparisons, there is a greater chance for **misclassification** of exposures or outcomes. Careful data handling and statistical techniques are required to manage this risk and ensure accurate results.

Both nested case-control and case-cohort studies provide the benefit of working within an existing cohort framework, ensuring a more efficient and often more reliable way to investigate risk factors for diseases. These designs are especially useful when the cost and time required to study an entire cohort are prohibitive, and they offer an effective balance between the thoroughness of cohort studies and the efficiency of case-control designs.

CHAPTER 4: MEASURING AND INTERPRETING RISK

Absolute vs. Relative Risk

Absolute risk and **relative risk** are two important ways to measure and understand the likelihood of developing a disease or health outcome. These measures help public health professionals, researchers, and clinicians interpret how risky a particular exposure or behavior is, and they guide decisions about interventions and treatments.

Absolute risk refers to the **actual probability** that an individual will develop a disease over a specific period. It is the simplest form of risk, calculated as the number of new cases of a disease divided by the total population at risk. Absolute risk gives a direct sense of how common a disease is in a particular group. For example, if 10 out of 1,000 people develop heart disease over the course of a year, the absolute risk of heart disease in that population is 1% per year.

Absolute risk is useful because it provides a **clear, concrete number** that reflects the likelihood of an event occurring. It answers questions like, "What is my risk of getting this disease?" or "How likely is it that someone in this population will develop this condition?" For example, if a doctor tells a patient that their absolute risk of developing lung cancer is 5% over the next 10 years based on their smoking history, the patient can understand that 5 out of every 100 people like them will likely develop the disease in that timeframe.

However, **relative risk** gives a different perspective. It **compares the risk of** disease between two groups—typically one that is exposed to a certain factor and one that is not. Relative risk is calculated by dividing the absolute risk in the exposed group by the absolute risk in the unexposed group. For example, if smokers have a 10% risk of developing lung cancer, and non-smokers have a 2% risk, the relative risk of lung cancer for smokers compared to non-smokers would be 5. This means smokers are five times more likely to develop lung cancer than non-smokers.

Relative risk is particularly valuable in **identifying the strength of an association** between an exposure and an outcome. It answers questions like, "How much more likely are smokers to get lung cancer compared to non-smokers?" or "What is the increased risk of heart disease in people with high cholesterol compared to those with normal cholesterol levels?"

While relative risk provides insight into the relationship between exposure and disease, it can sometimes be **misleading** without context. A large relative risk can sound alarming, but it may not reflect a high absolute risk. For example, if the absolute risk of a rare disease is 0.1% in the unexposed group and 0.3% in the exposed group, the relative risk would be 3, meaning the risk is three times higher for the exposed group. However, in absolute terms, the increase is only 0.2%, which may not be very concerning for most people.

Let's look at an example with numbers to clarify the difference between absolute and relative risk. Imagine two groups: one group of 10,000 people who regularly take a new medication and a second group of 10,000 people who don't take the medication. After a year, 200 people in the first group develop a particular side effect, while 100 people in the second group develop the same side effect.

- The **absolute risk** of the side effect for the first group (the medication group) is 200/10,000, or 2%.
- The **absolute risk** for the second group (the non-medication group) is 100/10,000, or 1%.

The **relative risk** comparing the two groups is 2% (in the medication group) divided by 1% (in the non-medication group), or 2. This means that people taking the medication are **twice as likely** to develop the side effect compared to those who don't take it.

In practice, it's important to consider both absolute and relative risk. If you only look at relative risk, a two-fold increase in risk may sound dramatic, but if the absolute risk is small (say, going from 1% to 2%), the actual increase in risk for any individual may not be as significant. On the other hand, if the absolute risk is already high (like going from 30% to 60%), a relative risk of 2 could represent a major concern.

When communicating risk to the public or patients, it's important to **present both absolute and relative risks** so that people can understand the real impact of the exposure or treatment. For instance, explaining that a medication doubles the risk of a side effect (relative risk) sounds concerning, but when you add that the absolute risk increases from 1% to 2%, it puts the information into perspective. Both measures are necessary for making informed decisions about health interventions and understanding the real-world implications of risk.

Odds Ratio and Risk Ratio

In epidemiology, **odds ratio (OR)** and **risk ratio (RR)** (also known as the relative risk) are two key measures used to compare the likelihood of an event or disease between two groups. Both help assess the strength of an association between an exposure and an outcome, but they are calculated differently and are used in distinct types of studies.

The **odds ratio (OR)** is primarily used in **case-control studies**, where researchers start with cases (people with the disease) and controls (people without the disease) and look back to assess their exposure history. The odds ratio compares the odds of exposure among the cases to the odds of exposure among the controls.

To calculate the odds, you divide the number of people exposed by the number of people not exposed. For example, in a study on lung cancer and smoking, you would calculate the odds of smoking among those with lung cancer (cases) and compare it to the odds of smoking among those without lung cancer (controls). The odds ratio tells you how much more likely (or less likely) someone with the disease is to have been exposed to the risk factor compared to someone without the disease.

For example, let's assume you conduct a study with 100 lung cancer patients (cases) and 100 people without lung cancer (controls). Out of the 100 cases, 80 are smokers, and 20 are non-smokers. Among the controls, 40 are smokers, and 60 are non-smokers. The odds of smoking in the cases are $80/20 = 4$, and the odds of smoking in the controls are $40/60 = 0.67$. The **odds ratio** is then $4/0.67 = 6$, meaning lung cancer patients are six times more likely to have been smokers than people without lung cancer.

The **risk ratio (RR)**, or relative risk, is used in **cohort studies** where researchers follow groups of people over time to see who develops the disease based on their exposure status. The risk ratio compares the **probability (risk)** of developing the disease in the exposed group to the risk in the unexposed group.

For instance, imagine a cohort study where you follow 1,000 smokers and 1,000 non-smokers over 10 years to see who develops lung cancer. If 50 smokers develop lung cancer and 10 non-smokers develop lung cancer, the risk of lung cancer in smokers is $50/1,000 = 0.05$ (or 5%), and the risk in non-smokers is $10/1,000 = 0.01$ (or 1%). The **risk ratio** is $0.05/0.01 = 5$, meaning that smokers have five times the risk of developing lung cancer compared to non-smokers.

While both measures describe the association between an exposure and an outcome, **risk ratios** are more intuitive because they directly express the probability of developing the disease. In contrast, **odds ratios** tend to overestimate the risk, especially when the outcome is common (greater than 10%). For rare outcomes, however, the odds ratio and risk ratio are similar.

Odds ratios are often used in case-control studies because the outcome (disease) has already occurred, and it's not possible to directly calculate risk. Instead, you work with the odds of exposure. Risk ratios, on the other hand, are used in cohort studies where researchers can observe how many people develop the disease over time, making it possible to calculate actual risks.

In **interpretation**, if the odds ratio or risk ratio is **greater than 1**, it suggests that the exposure increases the likelihood of the outcome. For example, an OR or RR of 2 means the risk is twice as high in the exposed group. If the value is **less than 1**, the exposure is associated with a reduced risk. If the OR or RR equals **1**, there is no association between the exposure and the outcome.

Attributable Risk

Attributable risk is a measure used in epidemiology to estimate the portion of a disease or health outcome that can be attributed to a specific exposure. It answers the question, "How much of the disease in the exposed group is due to the exposure?" This measure is crucial for understanding the **public health impact** of risk factors and for designing interventions aimed at reducing disease incidence.

Attributable risk is calculated by subtracting the incidence of disease in the unexposed group from the incidence of disease in the exposed group. This gives the additional risk that can be attributed to the exposure. In mathematical terms, attributable risk (AR) is:

$$AR = \text{Incidence in exposed group} - \text{Incidence in unexposed group}$$

For example, let's consider a cohort study investigating the relationship between smoking and lung cancer. Suppose the incidence of lung cancer among smokers is 200 per 100,000 people per year, and the incidence among non-smokers is 20 per 100,000 people per year. The attributable risk would be:

$$AR = 200 \text{ per } 100,000 - 20 \text{ per } 100,000 = 180 \text{ per } 100,000$$

This means that 180 cases of lung cancer per 100,000 people per year can be attributed to smoking. Essentially, if smoking were eliminated, you would expect 180 fewer cases of lung cancer per 100,000 people in the population.

Attributable risk is particularly useful for **quantifying the burden** of disease in an exposed population. Public health officials use this information to prioritize interventions. For instance, if the attributable risk of smoking for lung cancer is high, then policies aimed at reducing smoking rates (e.g., smoking cessation programs, tobacco taxes) could have a significant impact on lowering the incidence of lung cancer.

However, attributable risk doesn't tell you how strong the association between the exposure and disease is—**relative risk** or **odds ratio** does that. Instead, attributable risk measures the **absolute excess risk** due to the exposure. In other words, it provides a sense of how many cases of the disease could be prevented if the exposure were removed.

A related concept is **attributable risk percent (AR%)**, which expresses the attributable risk as a percentage of the total risk in the exposed group. AR% is calculated as:

$$AR\% = (\text{Attributable risk} / \text{Incidence in exposed group}) \times 100$$

Using the previous example of smoking and lung cancer, where the incidence of lung cancer in smokers is 200 per 100,000 and the attributable risk is 180 per 100,000, the AR% would be:

$$AR\% = (180 / 200) \times 100 = 90\%$$

This means that 90% of the lung cancer cases in smokers can be attributed to smoking. In other words, if smoking were eliminated, 90% of lung cancer cases in that population could be prevented.

Attributable risk can also be applied to **population-level analysis** through the concept of **population attributable risk (PAR)**. This measure estimates the amount of disease in the entire population (both exposed and unexposed) that is due to the exposure. PAR takes into account the **prevalence of exposure** in the population, making it a useful tool for understanding the overall impact of a risk factor on public health.

The formula for PAR is:

$$PAR = \text{Incidence in the total population} - \text{Incidence in the unexposed group}$$

For example, if the overall incidence of lung cancer in a population is 120 per 100,000, and the incidence among non-smokers is 20 per 100,000, the PAR would be:

$$PAR = 120 \text{ per } 100,000 - 20 \text{ per } 100,000 = 100 \text{ per } 100,000$$

This means that 100 cases of lung cancer per 100,000 people in the population can be attributed to smoking. Public health interventions targeting smoking would aim to reduce this burden.

Overall, attributable risk, attributable risk percent, and population attributable risk are key measures for understanding the impact of risk factors on disease in both specific groups and the broader population. These metrics help prioritize public health efforts and guide the development of policies aimed at reducing exposure to harmful risk factors.

Number Needed to Treat (NNT) and Number Needed to Harm (NNH)

Number Needed to Treat (NNT) and **Number Needed to Harm (NNH)** are important metrics used in clinical epidemiology to evaluate the effectiveness and potential risks of medical interventions. These measures provide insight into how many patients need to be treated with a particular therapy to achieve a beneficial outcome or, conversely, how many patients would experience harm from a treatment.

Number Needed to Treat (NNT)

Number Needed to Treat (NNT) refers to the number of patients who need to receive a specific treatment in order for one patient to benefit. It helps quantify the impact of an intervention by providing a concrete estimate of its effectiveness. NNT is particularly useful in helping clinicians weigh the benefits of a treatment against its potential costs or risks.

NNT is calculated using the **absolute risk reduction (ARR)**, which is the difference in the risk of an adverse outcome between the treatment group and the control group. ARR is derived from the **event rate** in both the treatment and control groups. The formula for NNT is:

$$NNT = 1 / ARR$$

Let's look at a practical example. Suppose a study on a new heart disease drug shows that 10% of patients in the control group experience a heart attack over a year, while only 5% of patients in the treatment group do. The ARR is 10% - 5% = 5% (or 0.05 when expressed as a proportion). The NNT would be:

$$NNT = 1 / 0.05 = 20$$

This means that 20 patients need to be treated with the drug to prevent one additional heart attack.

Interpreting NNT is straightforward. A lower NNT indicates a more effective treatment because fewer patients need to be treated for one to benefit. For example, an NNT of 5 means you only need to treat five people for one to benefit, while an NNT of 100 means you must treat 100 people to achieve the same benefit for one person. The closer the NNT is to 1, the more impactful the treatment.

Context matters when evaluating NNT. For life-saving interventions, an NNT of 100 may be considered worthwhile, especially if the condition being treated is severe. In contrast, for less critical conditions, an NNT of 20 or higher might be seen as less favorable, particularly if the treatment is costly or carries significant side effects.

It's important to note that NNT can change depending on the **baseline risk** of the population. If a patient population has a higher baseline risk for an adverse event, the absolute risk reduction may be larger, which could lower the NNT and make the treatment appear more effective. On the other hand, in populations with lower baseline risk, the same treatment might have a higher NNT, indicating it is less effective for that group.

Number Needed to Harm (NNH)

Number Needed to Harm (NNH) measures the **number of patients** that need to be treated with a specific intervention before one person experiences a harmful side effect or adverse outcome. NNH provides a way to quantify the risks associated with treatment and is particularly useful in assessing the safety of interventions.

NNH is calculated similarly to NNT, but instead of focusing on the reduction of adverse events, it looks at the **absolute increase in risk** of harm. The formula for NNH is:

$$NNH = 1 \text{ / absolute risk increase (ARI)}$$

To understand how NNH works, consider a drug that increases the risk of developing a serious side effect. If 1% of patients in the treatment group experience the side effect, compared to 0.2% in the control group, the ARI is 1% - 0.2% = 0.8% (or 0.008 as a proportion). The NNH would be:

$$NNH = 1 / 0.008 = 125$$

This means that 125 patients would need to be treated with the drug for one person to experience the harmful side effect.

Interpreting NNH works in the opposite direction from NNT. A **higher NNH** indicates a safer treatment because it suggests that harm is rare—many people must be treated before one person is harmed. A **low NNH**, on the other hand, signals a higher risk of harm, meaning fewer patients need to be treated for one to experience an adverse effect.

NNH is crucial for understanding the **risk-benefit balance** of a treatment. Even highly effective treatments with a low NNT must be considered carefully if they also have a low NNH, suggesting that they cause harm in a significant number of patients. For example, a treatment might have an NNT of 10, meaning it benefits one person for every 10 treated, but if the NNH is 15, meaning one person is harmed for every 15 treated, the overall safety profile of the treatment becomes a serious concern.

Balancing NNT and NNH

Clinicians often weigh NNT and NNH together to make informed decisions about treatments. Ideally, a treatment should have a **low NNT** (indicating effectiveness) and a **high NNH** (indicating safety). The greater the difference between NNT and NNH, the more favorable the risk-benefit ratio.

For example, if a treatment has an NNT of 50 and an NNH of 200, this suggests that for every 50 people treated, one person will benefit, and for every 200 people treated, one will be harmed. In this case, the treatment might be considered beneficial overall because the likelihood of harm is much lower than the likelihood of benefit.

However, when the NNT and NNH are close, the decision becomes more complex. If a treatment has an NNT of 10 but an NNH of 12, the likelihood of benefit is similar to the likelihood of harm. In such cases, clinicians must consider other factors, such as the severity of the disease, the potential impact of the harm, and the individual patient's preferences and risk tolerance.

Limitations of NNT and NNH

While NNT and NNH are valuable tools for decision-making, they are not without limitations. Both metrics depend on the **absolute risk reduction (ARR) or absolute risk increase (ARI)**, which can vary significantly across different populations. As mentioned earlier, the baseline risk of the population can change the NNT and NNH, meaning that the same treatment may appear more or less effective or risky depending on the group being studied.

Additionally, NNT and NNH are typically based on **short-term outcomes** and may not account for long-term benefits or harms. A treatment with a low NNT and a high NNH might look favorable in the short term, but if long-term risks or benefits emerge over time, these metrics may not capture the full picture.

NNT and NNH also do not account for the **severity** of the benefit or harm. A treatment that prevents a minor symptom (like a mild headache) but carries a risk of serious harm (like a life-threatening complication) would not be adequately evaluated by just looking at NNT and NNH. The **clinical significance** of the outcome must also be considered.

CHAPTER 5: DATA COLLECTION IN EPIDEMIOLOGY

Types of Epidemiologic Data Sources

Data collection is critical for understanding patterns of disease, identifying risk factors, and guiding public health interventions. Epidemiologists rely on various types of data sources to gather accurate, reliable information about health outcomes, exposures, and the populations affected. These data sources can be broadly classified into primary and secondary sources, each serving distinct purposes in public health research and practice.

Primary Data Sources

Primary data sources involve collecting new data directly from the population under study. These are tailored to the specific research questions or health issues being investigated, making them highly valuable for obtaining detailed and relevant information. Primary data collection methods include surveys, interviews, and direct clinical measurements.

1. **Surveys and Questionnaires**: Surveys are a widely used tool in epidemiology for gathering data on behaviors, exposures, and health outcomes from large populations. They can be administered in person, by phone, or online. Surveys like the **Behavioral Risk Factor Surveillance System (BRFSS)** in the United States collect data on lifestyle factors such as smoking, physical activity, and alcohol use. These surveys provide **self-reported** data, which can give insight into health behaviors and perceptions that might not be captured through medical records. However, they also carry the risk of **recall bias**, where participants may not accurately remember past behaviors or exposures.

2. **Interviews**: Interviews, whether structured or semi-structured, allow for more in-depth data collection. In structured interviews, a set list of questions is asked, while semi-structured interviews allow for more flexibility, giving respondents the chance to elaborate on their experiences. This method is particularly useful in qualitative epidemiology, where understanding the context around health behaviors or outcomes is important. For example, interviews might be used in studies exploring the social determinants of health, such as how economic or environmental factors affect access to healthcare.

3. **Direct Clinical Measurements**: Collecting **biological samples** or performing physical exams on study participants is another primary data source. Measurements like blood pressure, cholesterol levels, or blood sugar provide objective data that is not influenced by recall bias. This method is commonly used in **cohort studies**, where participants undergo regular health assessments over time. Direct measurements offer a clear

view of biological risk factors, making them essential for understanding diseases like cardiovascular conditions or diabetes.

Secondary Data Sources

Secondary data sources refer to data that have already been collected by other entities, such as government agencies, healthcare providers, or research institutions. These data are often gathered for purposes other than research, such as routine healthcare delivery or national statistics, but they are incredibly valuable for epidemiologists. Using secondary data can save time and resources, as researchers don't need to conduct new data collection. The most common secondary sources include vital statistics, disease registries, electronic health records, and surveillance systems.

1. **Vital Statistics**: Vital statistics include records of **births, deaths, marriages, and divorces**, often maintained by government agencies. **Death certificates**, in particular, are a key source of data for epidemiologists studying mortality rates and causes of death. These certificates typically include information on the primary cause of death as well as contributing factors, which can help identify patterns in mortality linked to specific diseases or health behaviors. For instance, increases in mortality from respiratory conditions might be tied to rising pollution levels, while changes in cardiovascular death rates could reflect shifts in diet and lifestyle.

2. **Disease Registries**: Disease registries are databases that systematically collect information on individuals diagnosed with specific diseases. For example, **cancer registries** track all cases of cancer diagnosed within a certain region. These registries offer valuable data on **incidence** (new cases) and **prevalence** (existing cases) of diseases, as well as information on treatment outcomes. Cancer registries, for example, can help track the success of treatment programs and identify trends in cancer incidence related to environmental exposures or genetic factors.

3. **Electronic Health Records (EHRs)**: EHRs are digital records of patients' medical histories, maintained by healthcare providers. EHRs include data on diagnoses, treatments, medications, and outcomes, making them a rich source of **longitudinal health data**. EHRs are particularly useful for tracking the long-term progression of chronic diseases like diabetes or hypertension. They also allow for the study of the effectiveness of various treatments in real-world settings, outside of controlled clinical trials. However, the use of EHRs in epidemiology can be complicated by issues of **data privacy** and **incomplete data**, as not all healthcare providers contribute to shared databases.

4. **Surveillance Systems**: Public health surveillance systems are designed to monitor and track diseases, injuries, and other health conditions in populations. These systems are crucial for **early detection of outbreaks** and for tracking the spread of infectious diseases. Examples include the **Centers for Disease Control and Prevention (CDC)** surveillance for flu

and the **Global Health Observatory** for tracking global health trends. Surveillance systems typically collect ongoing data on disease incidence, prevalence, and patterns, allowing public health officials to respond quickly to emerging threats like pandemics or the resurgence of previously controlled diseases.

Other Epidemiologic Data Sources

In addition to primary and secondary data, other sources such as **census data**, **environmental monitoring**, and **administrative data** are used in epidemiological studies.

1. **Census Data**: Census data provide demographic information, such as age, gender, race, income, and housing conditions. These data are critical for adjusting epidemiologic analyses to account for differences in population structure. For example, when studying disease incidence, it's important to adjust for age because many diseases are more common in older populations. Census data can also help identify social determinants of health, such as the relationship between income levels and disease prevalence.
2. **Environmental Monitoring**: Environmental data, such as air quality measurements, water quality assessments, and exposure to pollutants, are increasingly used in epidemiology. These data help link environmental exposures to health outcomes. For example, studies on asthma incidence often rely on air pollution data to explore how poor air quality contributes to respiratory conditions.
3. **Administrative Data**: Administrative data come from records kept by institutions like hospitals, insurance companies, or government agencies. These include **hospital discharge records**, insurance claims, and records of participation in public health programs. Administrative data are useful for evaluating the **utilization of healthcare services** and **treatment outcomes**. They can also help track trends in healthcare costs and access.

Overall, epidemiologists use a range of data sources to capture a full picture of health outcomes and risk factors. Whether through collecting new data or analyzing existing records, these sources help researchers uncover trends, identify risk factors, and guide public health interventions.

Surveys and Questionnaires

Surveys and questionnaires are essential tools in epidemiology for collecting data on health behaviors, exposures, and outcomes from large populations. They allow researchers to gather information directly from individuals, often about factors that are not easily measurable through medical records, such as lifestyle choices, self-reported health conditions, and social determinants of health. Surveys and questionnaires are particularly useful for epidemiological studies that focus on understanding risk factors for diseases, health disparities, and the prevalence of health behaviors.

A well-designed survey can reach thousands or even millions of people, providing epidemiologists with broad insights into public health. **Surveys** typically use structured, standardized questions that allow for easy comparison across individuals and populations. The **Behavioral Risk Factor Surveillance System (BRFSS)** is an example of a large-scale survey in the United States that collects data on health behaviors like smoking, physical activity, and alcohol consumption. This data helps public health officials track changes in health behaviors over time and identify high-risk populations that may need targeted interventions.

Questionnaires, which are often part of surveys, can be administered in different ways: **in person**, by **phone**, **mail**, or **online**. Each method has its advantages and challenges. In-person and telephone interviews allow researchers to clarify questions if participants are confused, which can improve the accuracy of responses. However, these methods are more expensive and time-consuming. Online and mailed questionnaires, on the other hand, are more cost-effective and can reach larger populations quickly, but they risk lower response rates and less control over how questions are understood by participants.

Question design is critical in epidemiology to ensure that the data collected is reliable and valid. Questions should be clear, concise, and free from ambiguity. **Closed-ended questions** (e.g., multiple choice or yes/no questions) are commonly used because they provide structured responses that are easy to analyze. For example, a question about smoking habits might ask, "Have you smoked cigarettes in the last 30 days? Yes/No." While closed-ended questions are easy to quantify, they may limit the depth of the responses. In contrast, **open-ended questions** allow respondents to elaborate on their answers, providing richer data, but these responses are more difficult to analyze and require more resources to process.

Surveys are especially helpful in **cross-sectional studies**, where data is collected at a single point in time to assess the **prevalence** of certain health conditions or behaviors. For instance, a cross-sectional survey on obesity might ask participants about their height, weight, dietary habits, and physical activity levels to estimate the prevalence of obesity in a particular community.

Surveys can also be used in **cohort studies** to follow participants over time. For example, participants in a long-term cohort study might complete periodic questionnaires about their diet, exercise, and mental health to track changes over several years. This longitudinal data helps researchers examine how certain behaviors or exposures relate to the development of diseases over time.

However, **bias** is a potential limitation in survey research. **Recall bias** can occur when participants are asked to remember past behaviors or exposures. For example, if a survey asks about alcohol consumption over the past year, some individuals may not accurately remember how much they drank. **Social desirability bias** is another concern, where participants may underreport behaviors that are socially frowned upon, such as smoking or overeating, and overreport positive behaviors like exercise. Carefully designed questions and **confidentiality assurances** can help mitigate these biases.

Another challenge is **low response rates**, particularly with mailed or online surveys. If certain groups of people are less likely to respond (e.g., people with low literacy or limited internet access), this can introduce **selection bias**, where the sample may not represent the broader population.

Despite these challenges, surveys and questionnaires remain valuable tools for collecting large-scale public health data. They are relatively inexpensive, flexible, and able to gather detailed information on a wide range of health-related topics, making them a cornerstone of epidemiological research.

Disease Registries

Disease registries are systematic collections of data about individuals diagnosed with specific diseases or conditions. These registries are crucial in epidemiology for monitoring disease incidence, prevalence, treatment outcomes, and survival rates over time. Registries often focus on chronic diseases like cancer, diabetes, cardiovascular conditions, and rare diseases, providing valuable data for research, public health planning, and policy-making.

A **cancer registry** is one of the most common types of disease registries. Cancer registries track information about patients diagnosed with various types of cancer, including tumor characteristics, stage at diagnosis, treatment methods, and survival outcomes. For example, the **Surveillance, Epidemiology, and End Results (SEER) Program** in the United States collects data on cancer incidence, treatment, and survival from a representative sample of the population. SEER data is widely used by researchers and policymakers to evaluate cancer trends, guide prevention efforts, and assess the effectiveness of screening programs.

Disease registries offer several key advantages for epidemiological research. First, they provide **longitudinal data** on patients, allowing researchers to follow individuals over time and track changes in health status, treatment outcomes, and survival. This type of data is critical for understanding the natural history of diseases and for evaluating the impact of treatments. For instance, a diabetes registry might track patients' blood sugar levels, medications, and complications over several years, providing insight into the effectiveness of different treatment approaches.

Registries also help identify **patterns of disease incidence and prevalence**. For example, a registry focused on cardiovascular disease might reveal that certain geographic regions have higher rates of heart disease, prompting further investigation into potential environmental or lifestyle factors contributing to the increase. Similarly, cancer registries can show trends in the incidence of specific cancers over time, helping to evaluate the effectiveness of prevention strategies like anti-smoking campaigns or vaccinations (e.g., for HPV).

Another significant use of disease registries is in **genetic epidemiology**. Registries that collect data on individuals with rare genetic diseases help researchers study how genetic mutations affect health outcomes and how these diseases are inherited within families. For example, registries tracking patients with **cystic fibrosis** or **Huntington's disease** can provide valuable data for understanding the genetic basis of these conditions and developing targeted treatments.

Disease registries also be important in **healthcare quality improvement**. By tracking treatment patterns and outcomes, registries allow healthcare providers to benchmark their performance against regional or national standards. For instance, a heart disease registry might track how quickly patients receive certain interventions (like angioplasty) after a heart attack and compare these metrics across hospitals. This information can be used to identify best practices and improve the quality of care.

While disease registries offer many benefits, they also have limitations. One challenge is the potential for **incomplete data**. Not all healthcare providers may contribute data to the registry, leading to gaps in coverage. For example, if a cancer registry only collects data from certain hospitals, it may miss cases diagnosed or treated elsewhere, leading to underestimates of disease incidence.

Data accuracy can also be an issue. Disease registries rely on healthcare providers to accurately report diagnoses, treatments, and outcomes. Errors in medical records or delays in reporting can affect the quality of the data. To address these issues, many registries implement rigorous **data validation** processes, such as cross-checking medical records or conducting audits to ensure the accuracy and completeness of the data.

Another limitation is **privacy concerns**. Disease registries collect sensitive personal health information, raising concerns about patient confidentiality. To protect patients' privacy, registries must comply with regulations like the **Health Insurance Portability and Accountability Act (HIPAA)** in the United States, which sets standards for protecting health information. Many registries use **de-identified data**, meaning personal information is removed to protect patient confidentiality while still allowing for valuable research.

Despite these challenges, disease registries are indispensable for understanding disease trends, improving treatment outcomes, and guiding public health interventions. They provide comprehensive, long-term data that helps drive advances in medical research and healthcare delivery.

Medical Records and Surveillance Systems

Medical Records and **Surveillance Systems** are two critical data sources in epidemiology, providing comprehensive information for studying disease patterns, risk factors, and health outcomes. These data sources help researchers and public health officials understand both individual and population health, guide interventions, and evaluate the effectiveness of treatments or policies.

Medical Records

Medical records are detailed documents maintained by healthcare providers that capture a patient's medical history, including diagnoses, treatments, procedures, medications, and health outcomes. These records are a valuable data source in epidemiology because they offer **longitudinal** information about patients over time, providing a full picture of their health journey. With the widespread adoption of **electronic health records (EHRs)**, data from medical records has become more accessible and structured, making it easier for epidemiologists to extract meaningful insights.

Epidemiologists use medical records to study **disease incidence** and **prevalence** in real-world clinical settings. For example, EHRs can track how many patients in a healthcare system are diagnosed with chronic conditions like diabetes or hypertension, allowing researchers to estimate the burden of these diseases within a population. This data helps public health officials allocate resources more effectively, directing care and prevention efforts to the most affected areas.

Cohort studies often use medical records to follow patients over time and examine the relationship between exposures (such as smoking or medication use) and outcomes (like cancer or heart disease). By linking patients' health records to other datasets, such as disease registries or death certificates, researchers can obtain more comprehensive information on long-term outcomes, including survival rates and cause of death.

A key advantage of using medical records is their ability to provide **objective clinical data**. Unlike self-reported surveys, which may be subject to recall bias, medical records contain data entered by healthcare providers during clinical visits. This includes **lab results, imaging studies,** and **medication prescriptions**, providing a more accurate representation of a patient's health status. For example, a study on asthma management might use EHRs to track patients' prescription refills for inhalers, assess their use of emergency services, and analyze lung function test results.

However, **data completeness** can be a challenge when using medical records in epidemiology. EHRs are primarily designed for clinical care, not research, so certain variables important to epidemiologists may be missing or inconsistently recorded. For instance, lifestyle factors like physical activity or diet, which are critical in understanding diseases like obesity or heart disease, may not be routinely documented in medical records. Researchers may need to supplement medical record data with information from other sources, such as surveys or patient interviews, to get a fuller picture of exposures.

Another issue is **coding accuracy**. Medical records rely on standardized diagnostic codes, such as those in the **International Classification of Diseases (ICD)** system, to categorize illnesses and treatments. Errors or inconsistencies in coding can affect the accuracy of epidemiological studies. For instance, a misclassification of diagnoses, such as confusing type 1 and type 2 diabetes, can skew the analysis of disease trends and risk factors.

Epidemiologists also face **data privacy** concerns when using medical records. Because these records contain sensitive personal information, access to them is tightly regulated. In the United States, **HIPAA (Health Insurance Portability and Accountability Act)** sets strict standards for the use and disclosure of protected health information. Researchers must often work with **de-identified** datasets, where personal identifiers such as names and addresses are removed, to minimize the risk of privacy breaches. However, this can limit the ability to link records to other data sources, such as employment or environmental exposure records, which may be important for understanding the full context of a patient's health.

Despite these challenges, medical records remain a vital resource in epidemiological research. They provide rich, longitudinal data that helps track disease patterns, evaluate treatment outcomes, and identify emerging health issues in populations.

Surveillance Systems

Surveillance systems are designed to continuously monitor health events and trends in populations. Unlike medical records, which are primarily for individual patient care, surveillance systems focus on **population-level** data collection and aim to detect, prevent, and control diseases. These systems are essential for identifying outbreaks, tracking the spread of infectious diseases, and monitoring chronic conditions and risk factors in real time.

One of the most well-known types of surveillance is **infectious disease surveillance**. Agencies like the **Centers for Disease Control and Prevention (CDC)** in the United States and the **World Health Organization (WHO)** operate surveillance systems to track diseases such as influenza, tuberculosis, and HIV. These systems collect data from multiple sources, including hospitals, laboratories, and clinics, to provide early warning signs of disease outbreaks. For example, during the COVID-19 pandemic, surveillance systems were critical in tracking the virus's spread, identifying hotspots, and guiding public health responses such as lockdowns, vaccination campaigns, and travel restrictions.

Surveillance systems are also used to monitor **non-communicable diseases** (NCDs) like heart disease, cancer, and diabetes. Systems like the **Behavioral Risk Factor Surveillance System (BRFSS)** collect data on health behaviors, such as smoking, alcohol use, and physical activity, that contribute to NCDs. By monitoring these behaviors over time, public health officials can assess the impact of prevention programs and adjust policies as needed. For instance, a rise in obesity rates detected by surveillance systems may prompt new public health campaigns promoting healthy eating and exercise.

Sentinel surveillance is a specific type of surveillance where select sites, known as sentinel sites, report data on specific diseases or conditions. These sites are typically chosen to be representative of a larger population, and their data helps detect trends and inform public health decisions. For example, a few hospitals may serve as sentinel sites for tracking seasonal flu activity, reporting the number of flu cases and the severity of symptoms. Sentinel surveillance is often more cost-effective than comprehensive surveillance because it focuses on a subset of the population, yet still provides insights into disease trends.

Surveillance systems can be **active** or **passive**. **Passive surveillance** relies on healthcare providers, laboratories, or individuals to report cases of disease voluntarily. For example, doctors might report cases of notifiable diseases like measles or tuberculosis to public health authorities. Passive surveillance is less resource-intensive but may lead to underreporting if cases are not consistently documented or reported. In contrast, **active surveillance** involves public health officials actively seeking out cases through direct contact with healthcare providers, reviewing medical records, or conducting surveys. Active surveillance is more resource-intensive but generally provides more accurate and complete data. It is often used during outbreaks to ensure that all cases are identified and managed quickly.

Surveillance systems have a key function in **evaluating the effectiveness of public health interventions**. By tracking disease incidence and prevalence over time, these systems can help determine whether vaccination programs, health education campaigns, or new treatments are reducing the burden of disease. For example, surveillance data on **HPV** infections and cervical cancer rates can show whether HPV vaccination programs are successfully preventing cancer in the population.

Another advantage of surveillance systems is their ability to provide **real-time data**. This is particularly important in rapidly evolving situations like infectious disease outbreaks. For example, during an Ebola outbreak, real-time surveillance data can help public health officials understand how the virus is spreading, where to focus resources, and how effective control measures are. In contrast, traditional epidemiological studies often take longer to collect and analyze data, making them less useful in urgent public health situations.

However, surveillance systems are not without challenges. One issue is the **timeliness** of data reporting. In passive surveillance systems, there may be delays in reporting cases, especially if healthcare providers are overwhelmed or under-resourced. This can hinder the early detection of outbreaks or trends. **Data quality** can also be a concern, as underreporting or misreporting can lead to inaccurate estimates of disease burden. Additionally, surveillance systems often require **significant infrastructure and funding** to maintain, especially in low-resource settings.

Despite these limitations, surveillance systems are a cornerstone of public health. They provide critical data for detecting outbreaks, monitoring chronic diseases, and evaluating the effectiveness of health interventions, ensuring that public health responses are based on accurate, up-to-date information.

CHAPTER 6: OUTBREAK INVESTIGATION

Steps in Outbreak Investigation

Outbreak investigations are essential in identifying the source and controlling the spread of diseases. When an outbreak is suspected, epidemiologists follow a series of well-defined steps to investigate and manage the situation effectively. Each step is important for collecting accurate information and implementing the right interventions.

1. Prepare for Fieldwork

Before heading into the field, the investigation team must prepare. This includes assembling the right personnel—often a mix of epidemiologists, laboratory scientists, and public health officials. The team gathers background information about the disease and ensures they have the necessary tools for investigation, such as questionnaires, lab supplies, and personal protective equipment (PPE). In some cases, they'll also need to review previous outbreak reports of the same disease to understand any similarities or recurring patterns.

2. Confirm the Outbreak

The next step is to confirm that an outbreak is actually occurring. An **outbreak** happens when there are more cases of a disease than expected in a given area or population over a specific period. To confirm this, investigators look at surveillance data or reports from healthcare facilities. Sometimes, what appears to be an outbreak is just an artifact of increased testing or changes in reporting practices. Investigators also verify the diagnosis by reviewing clinical data and, if necessary, collecting biological samples to confirm the presence of the pathogen.

3. Define and Identify Cases

Once the outbreak is confirmed, investigators establish a **case definition**. A case definition is a set of criteria used to identify who will be considered a case during the investigation. It typically includes **clinical features** (e.g., fever, diarrhea), **lab confirmation** of the disease (e.g., positive blood culture), and sometimes **time** and **place** constraints (e.g., cases in a particular city during a specific time frame). A precise case definition is critical for consistency and helps ensure that investigators focus only on relevant cases.

Once the case definition is in place, investigators begin **case-finding** by searching for people who meet the definition. This might involve reviewing medical records, interviewing healthcare providers, or contacting public health departments. Investigators may also ask patients about their symptoms, the onset date of the disease, and potential exposures. By gathering detailed information, they can start to build a clearer picture of how the disease is spreading.

4. Perform Descriptive Epidemiology

After identifying cases, investigators describe the outbreak in terms of **time**, **place**, and **person**. This is often done by creating an **epidemic curve** (epi curve), which shows the number of cases over time. The shape of the curve can help investigators understand whether the outbreak is a **point-source outbreak** (where exposure happens at a single time, like food poisoning) or a **propagated outbreak** (where the disease spreads from person to person).

Next, the investigators analyze the geographic distribution of cases. By mapping cases, they can spot clusters and identify areas with higher concentrations of disease, which may offer clues about the source. The "person" aspect looks at who is affected—whether certain age groups, genders, or occupations are more affected. For instance, if an outbreak disproportionately affects children, investigators might consider schools or daycares as potential sources.

5. Develop Hypotheses

Based on the descriptive data, investigators form hypotheses about the source of the outbreak and how it's spreading. These hypotheses are often based on common factors among cases. For example, if most cases are linked to a particular restaurant, investigators might hypothesize that contaminated food is responsible. Similarly, if an outbreak occurs among workers in a specific industry, the source could be related to a shared exposure at the workplace.

6. Evaluate Hypotheses

To test the hypotheses, investigators conduct **analytic studies**, typically using a case-control or cohort study design. In a case-control study, investigators compare people who got sick (cases) with those who didn't (controls), looking for differences in exposures. For instance, they might find that cases were more likely to have eaten a specific food item than controls, providing evidence that the food item is the source.

In a cohort study, investigators track an entire group (the cohort) over time to see who develops the disease. This design is particularly useful in outbreaks where all individuals were potentially exposed, such as a group of attendees at a wedding or conference. By comparing attack rates (the proportion of people who become ill) between those exposed and those unexposed, investigators can identify the likely source.

7. Implement Control and Prevention Measures

Even before the investigation is complete, it's often necessary to implement **control measures** to prevent further cases. If the source of the outbreak is strongly suspected or confirmed, action must be taken immediately. For example, if contaminated food is identified, the food is recalled, and the restaurant or processing facility is inspected. In the case of a waterborne outbreak, authorities might advise boiling water or shut down contaminated water systems.

Personal protective measures might also be recommended, such as vaccinations, antibiotics, or quarantining exposed individuals to stop the spread of disease. In some cases, public health advisories are issued to inform the public about protective actions they can take, like practicing good hygiene or avoiding certain areas.

8. Communicate Findings

Throughout the investigation, clear and effective communication is essential. Investigators must keep public health officials, healthcare providers, and the public informed about the outbreak's status and any new developments. They also need to communicate with other stakeholders, such as regulatory agencies or businesses affected by the outbreak.

At the end of the investigation, a final report is produced, documenting the findings, the source of the outbreak, and the control measures implemented. This report helps guide future responses to similar outbreaks and contributes to the overall body of knowledge in public health.

Identifying the Source of an Outbreak

In outbreak investigations, identifying the **source** of the outbreak is one of the most critical steps. Knowing the source allows public health officials to implement control measures that can stop the spread of the disease and prevent further cases. Epidemiologists use a combination of **descriptive data**, **analytic studies**, and **laboratory testing** to pinpoint where the outbreak began and how it spread.

The first step in identifying the source is to look at **patterns of disease**. Epidemiologists begin by creating an **epidemic curve (epi curve)**, which charts the number of cases over time. The shape of the curve can provide early clues about the type of outbreak. For instance, a **point-source outbreak**, where all cases result from a single exposure (like food poisoning at an event), tends to show a sharp, sudden increase in cases followed by a rapid decline. In contrast, **propagated outbreaks**, where the disease spreads from person to person, often show a more gradual rise in cases, with multiple peaks as the disease spreads through different waves.

Geographic data also help identify the source. Mapping cases by location often reveals **clusters** of illness, which can indicate the source of the exposure. If most cases are centered around a particular restaurant, workplace, or community, it's a strong indication that something in that environment could be causing the outbreak. **Spot maps** are often used in this process, marking the locations of cases on a geographic map to show the concentration of disease in specific areas. These maps can be refined further by looking at where individuals live, work, or spend time, offering more specific insights into where exposure likely occurred.

Next, epidemiologists conduct **analytic studies** to test hypotheses about the source. **Case-control studies** are commonly used in outbreak investigations. Investigators interview both individuals who got sick (cases) and those who didn't (controls), asking detailed questions about their behaviors, food consumption, places they visited, and other potential exposures. If a significantly higher proportion of cases report having eaten a particular food or visited a specific location compared to controls, it strengthens the hypothesis that this exposure is linked to the outbreak.

For example, during an E. coli outbreak linked to contaminated lettuce, investigators might find that 90% of the cases ate lettuce from a certain brand, while only 10% of the controls did. This clear difference between cases and controls points strongly to the contaminated lettuce as the likely source. Similarly, in waterborne outbreaks, epidemiologists might compare water consumption patterns between those who became ill and those who didn't, looking for common water sources.

In addition to case-control studies, **cohort studies** are another tool used to identify sources in specific settings where the exposure is known or suspected. For example, if an outbreak occurs among attendees of a wedding or conference, investigators can follow up with all participants to determine who got sick and who didn't. By comparing exposures—such as food or beverages consumed—they can identify the source of the infection.

Finally, **laboratory testing** is essential for confirming the source. If a particular food item, water supply, or environmental sample is suspected of causing the outbreak, samples are collected and tested for pathogens. For example, stool samples from patients can be analyzed to identify the causative agent, such as Salmonella or norovirus. Similarly, food samples from the suspected source can be tested for contamination. If the pathogen found in the food or water matches the pathogen found in the patients, it provides strong evidence that this is the source of the outbreak.

Genetic testing has become a valuable tool in modern outbreak investigations. Techniques like **whole-genome sequencing** allow scientists to compare the genetic profiles of bacteria or viruses from different patients and potential sources. If the pathogens share identical or nearly identical genetic sequences, it suggests they come from the same source. This method has been particularly useful in foodborne outbreaks, where pathogens can spread across large geographic areas, making it harder to trace back to the source.

Identifying the source of an outbreak requires a combination of careful data analysis, laboratory work, and on-the-ground investigation. By analyzing patterns of disease, conducting analytic studies, and confirming findings through lab testing, epidemiologists can determine where the outbreak began and stop its spread.

Field Epidemiology: Challenges and Strategies

Field epidemiology is the practice of investigating outbreaks and public health crises directly in the settings where they occur. Unlike controlled, laboratory-based studies, field epidemiology involves working in real-world environments, often in difficult and unpredictable conditions. While this work is critical for controlling the spread of disease and protecting public health, it presents several challenges. Field epidemiologists must adapt their methods and strategies to deal with these obstacles effectively.

One of the main challenges in field epidemiology is the **lack of infrastructure** in many outbreak settings. When investigating outbreaks in remote or low-resource areas, epidemiologists often lack access to basic tools like reliable electricity, internet access, or laboratory facilities. This can delay the collection and analysis of samples, making it harder to identify the source of an outbreak and implement control measures. In such cases, epidemiologists must rely on **mobile labs** or work with local facilities that may not have the same capabilities as larger, more advanced labs.

In addition, **data collection** can be difficult in field settings, particularly in areas where health records are poorly maintained or where people may be distrustful of outside investigators. For example, in regions with high levels of poverty or low literacy rates, epidemiologists may struggle to obtain accurate information from interviews or surveys. To overcome this, field epidemiologists often work closely with **local healthcare workers** who are familiar with the community and can help gather data more effectively. In some cases, using **simplified questionnaires** or **visual aids** can improve communication with participants.

Another challenge is **logistics**. Field epidemiologists often work in environments that are difficult to access, such as rural villages, conflict zones, or areas affected by natural disasters. Getting to these locations may require navigating poor roads, crossing rivers, or dealing with other physical obstacles. In some cases, travel restrictions due to security concerns or quarantines can further complicate the situation. To address these logistical hurdles, field epidemiologists need to be well-prepared, working with local authorities to arrange transportation and using **telecommunication tools** when in-person visits aren't possible.

Field epidemiology also presents **cultural and social challenges**. When investigating an outbreak, it's crucial to understand the **cultural context** of the affected population. Certain practices or beliefs can influence how people respond to illness or cooperate with public health officials. For instance, in the case of an Ebola outbreak in West Africa, traditional burial practices contributed to the spread of the virus because they involved close contact with the bodies of the deceased. Field epidemiologists had to work with local leaders and adapt their strategies to respect these customs while also promoting safer practices.

Building **trust** with the community is critical in field epidemiology, especially when dealing with sensitive issues like infectious diseases or vaccination campaigns. Misinformation or rumors about the causes of an outbreak can lead to resistance, making it harder to collect data or implement control measures. In some cases, there may be outright hostility toward public health workers, especially if the community feels they are being blamed for the outbreak or if they have had negative experiences with health interventions in the past. Field epidemiologists must engage with **community leaders** and **public health educators** to build trust and ensure cooperation.

In outbreak situations, **time pressure** is another significant challenge. Field epidemiologists often face the urgency of containing an outbreak before it spreads further. Delays in identifying the source of an outbreak or in implementing control measures can lead to a rapid escalation of cases. This requires epidemiologists to act quickly while maintaining **scientific rigor**. Developing **rapid response protocols**, such as pre-prepared investigation kits or communication templates, can help reduce delays.

Finally, working in the field can take a toll on the physical and mental health of the epidemiologists themselves. They may face long hours, harsh conditions, and emotional stress from witnessing suffering firsthand. **Burnout** is a real concern in field epidemiology, especially during prolonged outbreaks or when working in high-risk environments. To manage these stresses, field epidemiologists need strong **support networks**, both from their teams and from mental health professionals. Strategies like rotating fieldwork assignments and ensuring access to rest breaks can help mitigate these pressures.

Despite these challenges, field epidemiologists are essential for investigating outbreaks in real time. By adapting to difficult conditions, building trust with communities, and working closely with local authorities, they can respond effectively to emerging public health threats.

CHAPTER 7: SCREENING FOR DISEASE

Principles of Screening Programs

Screening programs are a cornerstone of public health. They are designed to detect diseases early in people who don't show symptoms yet, allowing for earlier treatment and potentially better outcomes. The effectiveness of a screening program depends on several key principles, which guide whether screening for a particular disease is appropriate and beneficial.

1. The Condition Should Be Important

A disease should have significant public health importance to warrant screening. This means the condition should have a high prevalence in the population or pose serious health risks, such as disability or death, if left untreated. Screening programs are often focused on diseases like cancer, cardiovascular conditions, or diabetes because they are common and have a substantial impact on public health. Screening for rare or less severe conditions may not be justified because the costs and resources involved in screening may outweigh the benefits for such a small or low-risk population.

2. There Should Be a Recognizable Latent or Early Symptomatic Stage

For screening to be effective, there needs to be a **preclinical phase** during which the disease is present but not yet causing symptoms. This period offers a window of opportunity for detection and early intervention. For example, cervical cancer often has a long preclinical phase where abnormal cells can be detected by a Pap smear before progressing to invasive cancer. If a disease progresses too rapidly or lacks a detectable early stage, screening won't be helpful because by the time the disease is detected, it might already be too late to intervene effectively.

3. The Screening Test Should Be Accurate

A good screening program relies on tests that are **sensitive** and **specific**. Sensitivity refers to the test's ability to correctly identify those who have the disease (true positives). If a test has high sensitivity, it minimizes the number of false negatives, meaning fewer cases of the disease will be missed. Specificity, on the other hand, measures the test's ability to correctly identify those who do not have the disease (true negatives). A highly specific test reduces the number of false positives, ensuring that healthy individuals are not mistakenly identified as having the disease, which could lead to unnecessary anxiety and further testing.

No test is perfect, and a balance between sensitivity and specificity is often needed depending on the disease and the consequences of missing or falsely identifying cases. For instance, breast cancer screening with mammograms tends to favor sensitivity to catch as many cases as possible, even if it means a few false positives.

4. The Test Should Be Acceptable and Safe

Screening tests need to be **safe**, non-invasive, and acceptable to the target population. If the test is too invasive, painful, or risky, people are less likely to participate, reducing the effectiveness of the screening program. For example, simple blood tests for cholesterol or glucose are widely accepted because they are minimally invasive and carry little risk. In contrast, a screening test that requires a surgical biopsy might not be suitable for routine population screening because of the risks involved.

In addition to safety, **cultural acceptability** is important. Some populations may be hesitant to participate in certain types of screening due to cultural beliefs or stigmas surrounding the disease. Public health officials need to ensure that the screening program respects these concerns and is designed in a way that encourages participation without alienating any group.

5. The Condition Should Have an Effective Treatment

Screening is only useful if there is an **effective treatment** available for those who are diagnosed with the disease. Early detection needs to lead to better outcomes for the patients. For example, early detection of high blood pressure can prevent heart attacks and strokes with proper treatment. In contrast, if a disease has no effective treatment or the early detection doesn't improve the prognosis, screening becomes less valuable. There's no benefit to detecting a disease earlier if nothing can be done to alter its course.

6. Screening Should Be Cost-Effective

The cost of running a screening program, including the cost of the test itself and follow-up care, should be justified by the benefits. This doesn't mean that every program must be inexpensive, but it should offer good value for the resources spent. A cost-effective screening program finds a balance between reducing the burden of disease and using healthcare resources efficiently.

For example, colon cancer screening with a fecal occult blood test (FOBT) is relatively inexpensive and can be done on a large scale, making it a cost-effective option. On the other hand, some advanced imaging tests may be too costly to justify their use in routine population screening, especially if the disease they detect is rare.

7. There Should Be a Defined Population to Screen

Screening programs work best when they target **high-risk groups** rather than the entire population. Screening everyone indiscriminately is inefficient and can lead to more false positives. For instance, mammography screening for breast cancer is typically recommended for women over a certain age (usually 40 or 50) because they are at a higher risk. Screening younger women, who have a lower risk of breast cancer, would likely yield more false positives and unnecessary follow-up procedures without offering much benefit.

In contrast, screening programs targeting **high-risk populations**—such as those with a family history of a certain disease or those exposed to specific environmental hazards—can be more effective and resource-efficient.

A well-designed screening program is built around these principles, ensuring that the benefits of early disease detection are balanced against the risks and costs.

Sensitivity, Specificity, and Predictive Values

In screening programs, **sensitivity** and **specificity** are critical measures of a test's performance, while **predictive values** help determine how useful the test is in practice. Together, these concepts help evaluate how well a screening test identifies those with and without a disease.

Sensitivity measures the test's ability to correctly identify those who have the disease. It is the proportion of true positives among all the people who actually have the disease. A highly sensitive test detects nearly all individuals who are diseased, minimizing the risk of false negatives. For example, if a screening test for cervical cancer has a sensitivity of 95%, it correctly identifies 95 out of 100 women who have the disease. However, it might still miss 5 women who do have it, which could delay necessary treatment.

A screening program designed to catch as many cases as possible, such as for diseases with severe consequences like HIV or cancer, prioritizes **high sensitivity**. Missing a case could have serious health consequences, so reducing false negatives is key.

Specificity, on the other hand, is the test's ability to correctly identify those who do not have the disease. It's the proportion of true negatives among all the people who are disease-free. A highly specific test minimizes the number of false positives. If a breast cancer screening method has a specificity of 90%, it correctly identifies 90% of women who do not have breast cancer, while the remaining 10% might be falsely labeled as positive, leading to unnecessary further testing or anxiety.

A balance between sensitivity and specificity is essential, and the trade-off depends on the disease and its consequences. For example, for diseases where a false negative is dangerous, such as HIV, sensitivity is prioritized. In contrast, for diseases where over-treatment could lead to harm, such as certain cancers, specificity might be given more weight.

In real-world settings, **predictive values** are crucial for interpreting screening test results. The **positive predictive value (PPV)** is the probability that a person with a positive test result actually has the disease. The **negative predictive value (NPV)** is the probability that a person with a negative test result is truly disease-free. Unlike sensitivity and specificity, which are inherent to the test, predictive values depend on the **prevalence** of the disease in the population being screened.

For instance, in populations where a disease is rare, the PPV will be lower because there are more false positives in relation to true positives. A breast cancer screening program in a younger population, where cancer is less common, might have many more false positives than a program in an older population. On the other hand, NPV tends to be higher in populations where the disease is rare, as most negative results are likely to be true negatives.

Understanding sensitivity, specificity, and predictive values helps public health officials and clinicians interpret the results of screening programs and make informed decisions about further diagnostic testing and treatments.

Screening Biases: Lead-Time, Length, and Selection Bias

Screening programs are subject to several **biases** that can distort the perception of a test's effectiveness. These biases can make a screening program seem more effective than it is, or they can mask potential shortcomings. The most common biases are **lead-time bias**, **length bias**, and **selection bias**.

Lead-time bias occurs when screening detects a disease earlier, giving the appearance of improved survival time, even though the patient's actual lifespan hasn't changed. The bias arises because screening finds the disease in its earlier stages, so the time between diagnosis and death appears longer simply because the diagnosis was made earlier. For example, if a cancer screening program detects tumors earlier, it may look like patients are living longer after diagnosis, but if the treatment doesn't actually prolong life, the extra time is just an illusion caused by detecting the disease earlier. Lead-time bias can make screening programs seem more beneficial than they truly are, especially if survival time is used as the main measure of success rather than overall mortality reduction.

Length bias relates to the fact that screening is more likely to detect slower-growing, less aggressive forms of a disease, which are more likely to be caught during routine screening intervals. Fast-growing, aggressive diseases are often missed by screening because they develop quickly between screening tests. For example, in breast cancer screening, slow-growing tumors might be detected more frequently because they stay detectable longer, while rapidly progressing tumors are missed until they cause symptoms. This creates the illusion that screening improves outcomes by detecting more treatable cases, when in reality, it is the nature of the tumors, not the effectiveness of the screening, that is responsible for the perceived benefit. Length bias can make it appear as though screening leads to better survival rates, even if it is not preventing deaths from the most aggressive cases.

Selection bias in screening arises when individuals who choose to participate in screening programs are not representative of the general population. Often, people who volunteer for screening are more health-conscious, have better access to healthcare, or may have a family history of the disease. These individuals might have different risk profiles compared to those who do not participate in screening, leading to skewed results. For example, if a colon cancer screening program is evaluated based on voluntary participants, it may appear highly effective, but this could be due to the fact that those who participate are healthier overall or more likely to engage in preventive health behaviors. This means that the apparent success of the screening program might not be generalizable to the broader population.

To mitigate these biases, researchers must carefully design screening trials and use appropriate outcome measures. **Randomized controlled trials (RCTs)**, where participants are randomly assigned to a screening group or a control group, can help reduce selection bias. Additionally, looking at **disease-specific mortality** rather than overall survival times helps minimize the impact of lead-time and length biases.

Evaluating the Cost-Effectiveness of Screening Programs

Evaluating the **cost-effectiveness** of screening programs is essential to determine whether they provide good value for public health resources. Screening programs aim to detect diseases early, which can lead to better outcomes and, in some cases, reduce long-term healthcare costs. However, not all screening programs are equally beneficial, and implementing a screening program comes with costs—both direct and indirect. Cost-effectiveness analysis helps public health officials decide whether a screening program is worth the investment.

1. Defining Costs and Benefits

To evaluate cost-effectiveness, the first step is to define the **costs** and **benefits** of the screening program. Costs include the expenses of conducting the screening tests, follow-up diagnostic procedures, treatment of the detected cases, and any management of false positives. Direct costs encompass the price of tests, healthcare personnel, equipment, and facilities. Indirect costs might include productivity losses due to missed work for appointments or long-term disability if the screening doesn't prevent disease progression.

On the benefits side, the goal of screening is to improve health outcomes, primarily by detecting diseases earlier when they are more treatable. Benefits are often measured in **quality-adjusted life years (QALYs)** or **life years gained (LYG)**. These metrics quantify both the quality and quantity of life added by an intervention. A screening program that prevents death from a disease or significantly improves quality of life for survivors offers a clear benefit.

When calculating cost-effectiveness, these costs and benefits are compared. The outcome of interest is often expressed as the **cost per QALY gained** or **cost per life year gained**. A lower cost per QALY indicates a more cost-effective screening program.

2. Costs of the Screening Test

The **cost of the screening test** itself is a major factor in determining whether a program is cost-effective. Low-cost, minimally invasive tests, such as **blood pressure checks** for hypertension or **cholesterol tests** for cardiovascular disease risk, are often more cost-effective because they can be administered easily to a large number of people. In contrast, screening tests that require specialized equipment or are more invasive, such as **colonoscopy** for colorectal cancer, tend to be more expensive, raising the overall cost of the program.

The **frequency of screening** also impacts cost. Annual screenings for a disease may be less cost-effective than screenings every five years, especially if the disease in question progresses slowly. Reducing the frequency of screenings without significantly compromising detection rates can be a way to improve cost-effectiveness.

3. Detecting Disease in Early Stages

A key assumption behind screening programs is that early detection leads to **better outcomes**. The earlier a disease is caught, the more likely it can be treated effectively, reducing future healthcare costs. For example, early-stage breast cancer detected through **mammography** can often be treated with less invasive therapies and has higher survival rates compared to cancer detected at later stages.

Cost-effectiveness improves when early detection leads to significant reductions in future healthcare expenses, such as the need for intensive treatments, hospitalizations, or surgeries. In cases like **cervical cancer screening** with **Pap smears**, detecting pre-cancerous lesions early can prevent the development of full-blown cancer, which would be far more expensive to treat and more harmful to the patient.

However, not all diseases benefit equally from early detection. Some cancers or chronic conditions may progress so slowly that treatment doesn't necessarily extend life or improve quality of life significantly, which reduces the cost-effectiveness of screening.

4. The Impact of False Positives and Negatives

Screening programs inevitably produce some **false positives** and **false negatives**, both of which have cost implications. A **false positive** occurs when the test suggests that a disease is present when it is not. False positives lead to **unnecessary follow-up tests**, procedures, and treatments, which increase costs without providing any health benefits. They can also cause anxiety and stress for patients. The more common false positives are, the less cost-effective the screening program becomes because of the added burden of unnecessary healthcare utilization.

False negatives, where the test misses the disease, can also affect cost-effectiveness, though in a different way. A false negative means a patient goes untreated, potentially leading to disease progression and more costly interventions down the line. While false negatives don't add immediate costs, they undermine the value of the screening program by allowing preventable cases to worsen.

5. Prevalence of Disease

The **prevalence** of the disease in the population being screened is a crucial factor in evaluating cost-effectiveness. Screening is more cost-effective in populations with **higher disease prevalence** because more true cases are detected relative to the costs of conducting the screening. For example, screening for **diabetes** in a population with a high prevalence of obesity and sedentary lifestyles is likely to be more cost-effective than screening in a population where these risk factors are less common.

In low-prevalence populations, the proportion of false positives tends to increase, leading to higher costs without significant health benefits. This is why many screening programs target specific high-risk groups rather than the general population. For example, **lung cancer screening** using low-dose CT scans is more cost-effective when limited to older adults with a history of heavy smoking, where the disease prevalence is higher.

6. Long-Term Outcomes and Cost Savings

Screening programs that prevent serious complications or death often lead to **long-term cost savings**. For instance, early detection and management of **hypertension** can prevent costly and severe outcomes like strokes or heart attacks. Similarly, screening for **colorectal cancer** and removing polyps during a colonoscopy can prevent cancer from developing, thus avoiding the high costs of cancer treatment.

However, the cost savings from preventing disease must be weighed against the upfront costs of screening and treatment of detected cases. In some cases, even if early detection increases the number of people receiving treatment, the overall healthcare costs may still be lower than treating advanced disease later. For example, the cost of treating early-stage prostate cancer may be less than the long-term costs of treating metastasized cancer.

7. Balancing Costs and Public Health Benefit

Ultimately, evaluating the cost-effectiveness of screening programs requires balancing the costs of the screening and follow-up care with the public health benefits. **Cost-effectiveness thresholds** are often used to guide decision-making. For example, if the cost per QALY gained is below a certain threshold (e.g., $50,000 per QALY in the United States), the program may be considered cost-effective. However, these thresholds can vary based on available resources, the severity of the disease, and societal values.

Overall, by focusing on high-prevalence populations, using cost-effective screening intervals, and minimizing unnecessary follow-up procedures, public health programs can make the most of their resources while providing significant health benefits to the population.

CHAPTER 8: BIAS AND CONFOUNDING IN EPIDEMIOLOGICAL STUDIES

Types of Bias: Selection, Information, and Recall Bias

In epidemiological studies, **bias** can distort the results and lead to incorrect conclusions. Bias refers to systematic errors in the design, conduct, or analysis of research that can produce misleading findings. It differs from random error, which occurs by chance. There are several types of bias that can occur in epidemiological research, with **selection bias**, **information bias**, and **recall bias** being among the most common. Understanding these biases is critical to interpreting study results accurately and ensuring the validity of conclusions drawn from epidemiological data.

Selection Bias

Selection bias occurs when the individuals included in a study are not representative of the population intended to be studied. This can happen if there is a systematic difference between those who are selected for the study and those who are not, leading to biased results. Selection bias affects both case-control and cohort studies, though it occurs in different ways depending on the study design.

In **case-control studies**, selection bias can happen if cases and controls are not selected from the same population. For instance, if cases are recruited from a hospital but controls are selected from a general population, the controls may not accurately reflect the population from which the cases arose. This creates a bias because the controls could differ systematically from the cases in ways unrelated to the exposure being studied.

In **cohort studies**, selection bias can occur if participants who are more likely to develop the outcome of interest are systematically more (or less) likely to be enrolled or followed up. For example, if people with higher health literacy are more likely to participate in a long-term study on cardiovascular disease, and these individuals also happen to have healthier lifestyles, the results may underestimate the true association between risk factors like smoking or diet and heart disease.

One common form of selection bias is **loss to follow-up** in cohort studies. If individuals who drop out of the study differ systematically from those who remain, this can bias the results. For instance, if people with poorer health outcomes are more likely to drop out of the study, the final analysis will skew toward a healthier population, leading to an underestimation of the risk associated with the exposure.

Another example is **healthy worker bias**, which occurs in occupational studies. Workers are generally healthier than the general population because people with severe illnesses or disabilities are less likely to be employed. Therefore, comparing health outcomes between workers and the general population can make the risks associated with workplace exposures seem smaller than they truly are.

Information Bias

Information bias occurs when there is a systematic error in how data on exposure or outcomes are measured. This bias can arise from inaccurate or incomplete data collection, misclassification of exposures or outcomes, or differences in how information is gathered for different study groups. Information bias can occur in both case-control and cohort studies and often leads to **misclassification bias**.

Misclassification occurs when individuals are incorrectly categorized regarding their exposure status or disease outcome. It can be **differential** or **non-differential**. **Non-differential misclassification** happens when the misclassification of exposure or outcome occurs equally across all study groups. This type of bias tends to dilute the association between the exposure and outcome, making it harder to detect a true effect. For example, if a study on lung cancer misclassifies both smokers and non-smokers equally, it will likely weaken the association between smoking and lung cancer.

Differential misclassification, on the other hand, occurs when the error in classification is different for the exposed and unexposed groups or for cases and controls. This can either exaggerate or mask the true association between exposure and outcome. For instance, if cases of a disease are more thoroughly investigated than controls, there is a greater chance that subtle exposures will be detected in the cases, leading to an inflated estimate of the association between the exposure and the disease.

One common form of information bias is **observer bias**, which occurs when researchers' knowledge of participants' exposure status influences how they record or interpret data. For example, in a study of asbestos exposure and lung disease, if a researcher is aware that a participant worked with asbestos, they may be more likely to record respiratory symptoms as significant, even if similar symptoms in an unexposed person would be considered minor.

Interviewer bias is another type of information bias that can occur during the data collection process. If interviewers know whether participants are cases or controls, they might phrase questions differently or probe more deeply with cases, which could lead to differential reporting of exposures.

Recall Bias

Recall bias is a specific type of information bias that occurs in **retrospective studies**, particularly in case-control studies. It arises when there are differences in how participants remember and report past exposures. People with a disease (cases) are often more likely to recall exposures or events from the past because they may search for a reason or explanation for their illness. This heightened awareness can lead to **over-reporting** of exposures, while individuals without the disease (controls) might be less motivated to recall details about their past behaviors or exposures, leading to **under-reporting**.

For example, in a case-control study investigating the link between pesticide exposure and Parkinson's disease, individuals diagnosed with Parkinson's might be more likely to remember and report pesticide exposure compared to healthy controls, simply because they are more attuned to potential causes of their condition. This would result in an overestimation of the association between pesticide exposure and Parkinson's disease.

Recall bias can also affect **prospective studies** if participants' knowledge of their exposure status influences how they report symptoms or outcomes over time. For instance, in a study examining the long-term effects of a specific medication, participants who know they are taking the drug might be more likely to report side effects, even if those effects are not objectively related to the medication.

Minimizing recall bias can be challenging, but there are strategies to reduce its impact. One approach is to use **standardized questionnaires** with carefully designed questions that prompt participants to recall events as accurately as possible. Additionally, using **objective measures** of exposure, such as medical records or environmental monitoring data, can help avoid reliance on participants' memories.

Minimizing Bias in Epidemiological Studies

To minimize the impact of **selection, information, and recall biases**, careful study design and data collection procedures are crucial. Randomization, where appropriate, can reduce selection bias by ensuring that the exposed and unexposed groups are comparable. **Blinding** interviewers and participants to the study hypothesis or exposure status can help reduce information and interviewer biases. Using **standardized data collection methods** and relying on objective data sources where possible also help minimize misclassification and recall errors.

Each of these biases can distort study results, but by recognizing their potential and taking steps to address them, epidemiologists can improve the accuracy and reliability of their research. Understanding the types of bias that can occur in epidemiological studies allows for better interpretation of the findings and more informed decisions about public health interventions and policies.

Confounding Factors and Control Methods

In epidemiological studies, **confounding factors** can distort the relationship between an exposure and an outcome, leading to incorrect conclusions. A confounder is a variable that is related to both the exposure and the outcome but is not on the causal pathway. For example, in a study investigating the relationship between alcohol consumption and heart disease, **age** could be a confounding factor. Older individuals might drink more alcohol and are also at higher risk for heart disease. Without accounting for age, it could appear that alcohol is more strongly related to heart disease than it actually is.

Confounding factors make it difficult to determine whether the observed effect is truly due to the exposure being studied or whether it is influenced by other variables. Therefore, identifying and controlling for confounders is critical in producing accurate, reliable results in epidemiology.

There are several methods for **controlling confounding** in epidemiological studies:

1. **Randomization**: In **randomized controlled trials (RCTs)**, participants are randomly assigned to different groups, which helps evenly distribute both known and unknown confounders across the study groups. This method is the most effective way to eliminate confounding, but it's only feasible in experimental studies, not observational ones. Randomization ensures that any differences in outcomes between the groups can be attributed to the exposure rather than confounders.
2. **Restriction**: This method involves limiting the study population to people who fall within a certain range for the confounding variable. For example, if age is a confounder, the study might include only participants in a narrow age range, such as 30 to 40 years old. By doing this, the potential influence of age on the relationship between the exposure and outcome is minimized. However, restriction can reduce the generalizability of the study's findings since the results may not apply to people outside the restricted group.
3. **Matching**: In **case-control studies**, researchers can match cases and controls based on the confounding variable. For example, if gender is a potential confounder in a study on smoking and lung cancer, cases (people with lung cancer) can be matched to controls (people without lung cancer) based on gender. This ensures that the comparison between cases and controls isn't biased by differences in gender distribution. Matching is useful but can be time-consuming, and it only controls for the confounders that are specifically matched.
4. **Stratification**: **Stratification** involves dividing the study population into subgroups (strata) based on the confounding variable and analyzing each subgroup separately. For example, in a study on the link between physical activity and diabetes, participants could be stratified by age groups (e.g., 20-30, 30-40) to see if the association between physical activity and diabetes is consistent across different age categories. By stratifying,

researchers can control for the confounding effect of age and compare results across similar groups.

5. **Multivariable Adjustment**: One of the most common methods for controlling confounding is **multivariable adjustment**, typically done through statistical techniques like **multivariable regression analysis**. In this method, the outcome is modeled as a function of the exposure and multiple confounders. For example, in a study on diet and heart disease, variables like age, gender, smoking status, and exercise level can be included in the regression model to adjust for their potential confounding effects. This method allows researchers to isolate the independent effect of the exposure on the outcome.

Effect Modification and Interaction

Effect modification (also known as interaction) occurs when the relationship between an exposure and an outcome differs depending on the level of another variable, known as the **effect modifier**. In other words, the effect of the exposure on the outcome is modified by the presence or level of another factor. Recognizing effect modification is important because it highlights that the exposure-outcome relationship is not uniform across all subgroups of the population, and it provides insights into which populations may be most affected by a particular exposure.

To understand effect modification, consider a study on the relationship between smoking and lung cancer. If the effect of smoking on lung cancer risk is stronger in people with a family history of lung cancer compared to those without a family history, then family history is acting as an effect modifier. In this case, smoking increases the risk of lung cancer more for individuals with a genetic predisposition.

Effect modification is different from confounding. While confounding creates a false impression of an association, effect modification is a real phenomenon that provides valuable information about how different factors influence health outcomes. Detecting effect modification helps public health officials target interventions to the groups most at risk.

Identifying effect modification involves examining whether the association between the exposure and outcome differs across levels of a third variable. This can be done by **stratifying** the data by the potential effect modifier and looking at the exposure-outcome relationship in each stratum. If the strength or direction of the association differs significantly between strata, effect modification is present.

For example, imagine a study on the effect of exercise on heart disease risk, with gender as a potential effect modifier. If the protective effect of exercise is much stronger in women than in men, gender is an effect modifier. The researchers would stratify the analysis by gender, showing different risk estimates for men and women.

Effect modification can be **additive** or **multiplicative**:

1. **Additive effect modification** occurs when the combined effect of two variables is greater than the sum of their individual effects. For example, if both smoking and asbestos exposure increase the risk of lung cancer, the combined risk for people exposed to both might be higher than just adding the two individual risks together. This indicates that the interaction between smoking and asbestos is amplifying the risk more than expected.
2. **Multiplicative effect modification** occurs when the joint effect of two variables is greater than their individual effects multiplied together. For instance, if taking a certain medication increases the risk of a side effect, and a genetic mutation also increases that risk, the combined effect of both the medication and the mutation could be higher than simply multiplying the individual risks. Multiplicative effect modification suggests that the exposure and modifier are working together in a synergistic way to produce a much greater effect.

Statistical interaction tests are often used to detect effect modification. In regression models, an **interaction term** is included to test whether the effect of the exposure on the outcome differs across levels of the potential effect modifier. If the interaction term is statistically significant, it indicates the presence of effect modification.

Effect modification is important for **targeted interventions** and personalized medicine. By identifying subgroups where the exposure-outcome relationship is stronger or weaker, public health strategies can be tailored to specific populations. For instance, if older adults are more affected by a particular environmental exposure, interventions might focus on reducing that exposure in senior populations. Similarly, effect modification findings can guide clinicians in choosing the best treatment for individual patients based on their risk profile.

CHAPTER 9: CAUSALITY IN EPIDEMIOLOGY

Bradford Hill Criteria for Causation

In epidemiology, determining whether a relationship between an exposure and an outcome is **causal** is a critical challenge. Sir Austin Bradford Hill, a British epidemiologist, outlined nine criteria to help researchers evaluate whether an observed association is likely to be causal. These are known as the **Bradford Hill criteria** for causation. These criteria do not provide absolute proof of causality but guide researchers in assessing the strength of the evidence.

1. Strength of Association

The stronger the association between the exposure and the outcome, the more likely it is that the relationship is causal. For instance, in studies of smoking and lung cancer, smokers were found to have much higher rates of lung cancer compared to non-smokers, with relative risks often above 10. A strong association like this is less likely to be explained by bias or confounding. However, weaker associations can still be causal, but they require more evidence to rule out other explanations.

2. Consistency

If multiple studies, conducted by different researchers, in different settings, consistently find the same association, it strengthens the case for causality. For example, the relationship between asbestos exposure and lung cancer has been observed across various studies worldwide, reinforcing the likelihood that asbestos is a cause of lung cancer. Consistency across populations, time periods, and study designs increases confidence that the observed effect is not due to chance or bias.

3. Specificity

Specificity refers to the idea that a single exposure should lead to a specific outcome. For instance, smoking is specifically linked to lung cancer, though it also causes other diseases. While specificity is useful, it is not a strict requirement for causality because many exposures can lead to multiple outcomes, and many diseases have multiple causes. For example, physical inactivity is associated with a range of diseases like heart disease, diabetes, and obesity.

4. Temporality

Temporality is one of the most critical criteria for causality: the exposure must occur before the outcome. If the outcome appears before the exposure, the relationship cannot be causal. For example, if a person is diagnosed with lung cancer and only begins smoking after the diagnosis, smoking cannot be considered the cause. Temporality is often easier to establish in **cohort studies** where individuals are followed over time from exposure to outcome.

5. Biological Gradient

This criterion refers to the presence of a **dose-response relationship**, where increasing levels of exposure lead to increasing risks of the outcome. For example, the risk of lung cancer increases with the number of cigarettes smoked per day or the number of years a person has smoked. The biological gradient supports the argument for causality because it suggests a direct relationship between the exposure and the risk of disease. However, the absence of a dose-response relationship does not rule out causality, as some exposures may have threshold effects, where the disease occurs only after a certain level of exposure.

6. Plausibility

A causal relationship is more likely if there is a **biological mechanism** that explains how the exposure leads to the outcome. For example, it is biologically plausible that smoking causes lung cancer because tobacco smoke contains carcinogens that damage lung cells. However, lack of detailed knowledge about the biological mechanism does not rule out causality. In some cases, we may observe a strong association before fully understanding the underlying mechanisms, as was initially the case with smoking and lung cancer.

7. Coherence

Coherence means that the association between exposure and outcome should be consistent with existing knowledge, including laboratory findings and biological evidence. If epidemiological findings align with what is known from experimental biology or other fields, it strengthens the argument for causality. For instance, the association between asbestos and lung cancer is coherent with laboratory studies showing that asbestos fibers can cause lung damage and cellular mutations.

8. Experiment

The strongest evidence for causality often comes from **experimental studies**, such as randomized controlled trials (RCTs). In RCTs, exposure is randomly assigned, reducing the risk of confounding. For ethical reasons, many exposures cannot be tested experimentally in humans, but natural experiments or interventions can provide useful evidence. For example, public health interventions to reduce air pollution in certain regions can be followed by decreases in respiratory diseases, supporting the idea that air pollution causes these diseases.

9. Analogy

Finally, analogy refers to the use of similar known associations to argue for causality. If an exposure causes one disease, it might also cause a related disease. For instance, because smoking is known to cause lung cancer, it is plausible that other forms of tobacco use, like chewing tobacco, could cause oral cancer. Analogies help when direct evidence is weaker but related evidence is strong.

Association vs. Causation

Association and **causation** are distinct concepts that often get confused. An **association** means that two variables are related in some way. For example, an increase in one variable might be associated with an increase (or decrease) in another. However, association alone does not imply that one variable **causes** the other. Establishing **causation**—the idea that changes in one variable directly result in changes in another—requires a deeper analysis and a more rigorous set of evidence.

An **association** between two variables can be observed when the occurrence of one variable is linked to the occurrence of another. For example, studies may show that people who drink more coffee are less likely to develop type 2 diabetes. This is an association because both variables—coffee consumption and the incidence of diabetes—are related. But this doesn't mean coffee **causes** a lower risk of diabetes. There could be other factors at play, such as lifestyle differences between coffee drinkers and non-drinkers, or genetic factors that influence both coffee consumption and diabetes risk.

Associations can be **positive** or **negative**. In a positive association, both variables move in the same direction: as one increases, the other also increases. For example, the association between cigarette smoking and lung cancer is positive because more smoking is linked to higher rates of lung cancer. In a **negative association**, one variable increases as the other decreases. For example, there's a negative association between exercise and heart disease: as physical activity increases, the risk of heart disease tends to decrease.

Correlation and Confounding

Sometimes, associations are purely **correlational** and do not imply a direct cause-and-effect relationship. For instance, the number of ice cream sales and the number of drownings tend to increase in the summer months. While these two variables are correlated, eating more ice cream doesn't cause drowning. Instead, the underlying factor is the warmer weather, which increases both ice cream consumption and swimming-related accidents. This is an example of a **confounding factor**—a third variable that affects both the exposure and the outcome, creating a misleading association.

Confounding is one of the most common reasons why association does not imply causation. A **confounder** is a variable that is related to both the exposure and the outcome but is not on the causal pathway. For example, in studies examining the relationship between alcohol consumption and heart disease, **age** might be a

71

confounding factor. Older individuals may drink more alcohol and also have a higher risk of heart disease, but the relationship between alcohol and heart disease might disappear once age is accounted for. Confounders can distort the observed association, making it difficult to determine if the exposure is truly causing the outcome.

Causation: Establishing a Cause-and-Effect Relationship

In contrast to association, **causation** implies that changes in one variable lead to changes in another. Establishing causality requires more rigorous evidence and often involves ruling out alternative explanations like confounding. There are several ways to determine whether an observed association is likely to be causal, the most prominent being the **Bradford Hill criteria**, which provide a framework for assessing whether an exposure is likely to cause an outcome.

One of the key criteria for establishing causation is **temporality**. This means the exposure must occur before the outcome. For example, to say that smoking causes lung cancer, we need evidence that people started smoking before they developed cancer. If people began smoking after their cancer diagnosis, smoking clearly wouldn't be the cause.

Another important criterion is **strength of association**. Strong associations—where exposure is very clearly linked to the outcome—are more likely to be causal. For example, the relative risk of lung cancer in smokers compared to non-smokers is very high, providing strong evidence that smoking is a cause of lung cancer.

Causality in Observational Studies vs. Experimental Studies

One of the major challenges in epidemiology is determining causality in **observational studies**. Observational studies, such as **cohort** or **case-control** studies, don't involve direct manipulation of the exposure. Instead, researchers observe the natural occurrence of exposures and outcomes in populations. These studies can identify associations but are more vulnerable to confounding and bias, making it harder to establish causality.

In contrast, **randomized controlled trials (RCTs)** are considered the gold standard for determining causality. In RCTs, participants are randomly assigned to different groups, ensuring that the exposure is the only difference between the groups. This method minimizes confounding and bias, allowing researchers to draw stronger conclusions about causality. For example, an RCT might randomly assign participants to take a new drug or a placebo, and the difference in outcomes between the groups can be more confidently attributed to the drug.

However, not all exposures can be tested in experimental studies due to ethical or practical limitations. For example, it would be unethical to randomly assign people to smoke cigarettes to study the effects on lung cancer. Therefore, epidemiologists often rely on well-conducted observational studies and use criteria like the Bradford Hill criteria to infer causality.

Reverse Causality and Bidirectional Relationships

Another issue in understanding association and causation is **reverse causality**, where the outcome influences the exposure rather than the other way around. For instance, in studies on obesity and depression, it might be that depression leads to weight gain (due to emotional eating or reduced physical activity), rather than obesity causing depression. In this case, reverse causality complicates the understanding of which factor is driving the association.

Sometimes, the relationship between variables can be **bidirectional**, meaning that both variables influence each other. For example, poor mental health might lead to smoking, while smoking can worsen mental health. Understanding whether a relationship is causal, and in which direction, is important for designing effective public health interventions.

Direct and Indirect Causation

In epidemiology, **causation** can be **direct** or **indirect**, depending on how an exposure influences an outcome. Understanding this distinction helps researchers trace the pathways through which health effects arise, which is important for designing effective interventions.

Direct Causation

Direct causation occurs when an exposure directly leads to an outcome without any intermediate steps or variables. In other words, there is a **straightforward cause-and-effect relationship** between the exposure and the outcome. For example, exposure to a pathogen like the **influenza virus** directly causes the disease **influenza**. There is no need for an intermediary factor to explain why exposure to the virus leads to the development of the disease.

Direct causation is often easier to identify because the relationship between the exposure and the outcome is immediate and apparent. For example, ingesting a toxic substance such as **cyanide** causes poisoning and death through a direct biological mechanism. In these cases, there is a clear pathway from exposure to outcome that doesn't involve additional factors or processes.

However, not all relationships in epidemiology are as straightforward as direct causation. Many health outcomes are influenced by complex interactions between multiple factors, which leads us to the concept of **indirect causation**.

Indirect Causation

Indirect causation occurs when the exposure affects the outcome through one or more intermediary steps or variables, known as **mediators**. In these cases, the relationship between the exposure and the outcome is more complex, and the effect is not immediate. For example, **poverty** can indirectly lead to poor health outcomes. Poverty may reduce access to nutritious food, quality healthcare, and safe living conditions, all of which are intermediary factors that increase the risk of diseases like diabetes or cardiovascular disease. Poverty doesn't directly cause these diseases, but it influences other factors that contribute to their development.

Another classic example of indirect causation is the link between **smoking** and **heart disease**. Smoking doesn't directly cause heart disease in the same way it causes lung damage through the inhalation of harmful chemicals. Instead, smoking raises blood pressure, increases inflammation, and promotes the buildup of fatty deposits in arteries, which in turn increases the risk of heart disease. The relationship between smoking and heart disease is mediated by these biological processes, making it an example of indirect causation.

Pathways of indirect causation are common in **chronic diseases** and other complex health outcomes. For example, **obesity** indirectly contributes to many health problems, such as diabetes and cancer. The excess weight doesn't cause cancer directly but leads to other changes, like insulin resistance, chronic inflammation, and hormonal imbalances, that promote the development of cancer.

Identifying and Addressing Indirect Causation

Recognizing indirect causation is important because it helps epidemiologists identify potential points for intervention. In cases of direct causation, the intervention is obvious: remove the exposure, and the outcome is prevented. For instance, preventing the spread of malaria by eliminating mosquito populations directly addresses the cause of the disease.

With indirect causation, interventions often target the **intermediary factors**. For example, to reduce the health impacts of poverty, public health interventions might focus on improving access to healthcare, promoting healthier diets, or providing safe housing. In the case of smoking and heart disease, interventions might focus on reducing blood pressure or improving diet and exercise habits in addition to encouraging smoking cessation.

Causal Pathways

In many cases, **direct and indirect causation** can work together in what are called **causal pathways**. A single exposure may lead to a sequence of direct and indirect effects, all contributing to the final outcome. Understanding these pathways is key for designing effective interventions. For example, in the **causal pathway** between smoking and lung cancer, the direct effect of smoking is the introduction of carcinogens into the lungs, which damages lung cells. This is a direct cause of cellular mutations leading to cancer. However, smoking may also indirectly affect lung health through chronic inflammation or immune system suppression, both of which contribute to the overall cancer risk.

By mapping out these pathways, epidemiologists can identify multiple points for intervention. Addressing both direct and indirect causes allows for a **multifaceted approach** to prevention. For example, reducing smoking rates is a direct intervention, but targeting inflammation or promoting lung health through public health campaigns may address some of the indirect mechanisms that contribute to the same disease outcome.

Intervening on Indirect Causes

Public health interventions often focus on indirect causes because they can be more feasible or practical to address than direct causes. For instance, while the direct cause of **diabetes** may be insulin resistance or pancreatic dysfunction, it might be more effective to intervene by addressing **dietary habits**, physical activity, or weight management—factors that indirectly influence the development of diabetes.

In some cases, focusing on **social determinants of health**, like improving education or access to healthcare, can indirectly reduce the prevalence of many diseases. By tackling these upstream factors, epidemiologists and public health officials can create broad, long-term improvements in population health, even if they're not directly eliminating the specific biological cause of a disease.

The Complexity of Indirect Causation

One challenge in dealing with indirect causation is the complexity of identifying all the relevant mediating factors. For instance, the effects of **stress** on health can be indirect and multifaceted. Chronic stress doesn't directly cause heart disease, but it can lead to unhealthy behaviors such as overeating, smoking, and physical inactivity. Stress also affects physiological systems by increasing blood pressure and promoting inflammation, which in turn increases heart disease risk. Understanding these indirect pathways is essential for designing effective interventions that go beyond merely treating the symptoms and aim to alter the underlying causes.

Temporal Sequence in Causal Relationships

Establishing **temporality**, or the correct **temporal sequence** between an exposure and an outcome, is critical for determining **causality**. Temporality means that the exposure must occur before the outcome for the relationship to be causal. Without proper temporal sequence, an observed association between two variables could be misleading or simply non-causal.

To illustrate, imagine a study examining whether air pollution causes asthma. For air pollution to be considered a causal factor, it must be shown that individuals were exposed to polluted air **before** they developed asthma. If asthma cases occurred before the individuals were exposed to air pollution, we could not reasonably claim that pollution caused the asthma. Establishing the correct sequence of events is the first requirement in demonstrating causality.

Importance of Temporal Sequence

Temporality is the only **Bradford Hill criterion** that is absolutely necessary for causality. Without it, any observed association may be spurious. For instance, reverse causality—a situation in which the outcome actually influences the exposure —can confuse the interpretation of study findings. An example of reverse causality would be a study that shows an association between sedentary behavior and obesity but fails to account for the fact that obesity may lead people to be more sedentary, not the other way around.

Cohort studies are particularly useful for establishing temporality because they follow individuals over time. Participants are classified by exposure status at the beginning of the study and then followed to see if they develop the outcome. For example, a cohort study on smoking and lung cancer would begin by identifying who smokes and who does not. The participants would then be tracked over several years to see if smokers develop lung cancer at a higher rate than non-smokers. This design ensures that smoking is documented before lung cancer occurs, satisfying the criterion of temporality.

In **case-control studies**, temporality can be more challenging to establish because the outcome has already occurred when the study begins. Researchers work backward, identifying cases (people who have the disease) and controls (people who do not) and then attempting to reconstruct past exposures. While this design can uncover associations, proving that the exposure preceded the disease often relies on accurate recall of past behaviors, which introduces potential biases, such as recall bias.

Temporality in Chronic vs. Acute Conditions

The role of temporality can differ depending on whether the disease is chronic or acute. In **acute diseases**, such as foodborne illnesses, the temporal relationship is usually clearer because the time between exposure (e.g., eating contaminated food) and the outcome (e.g., food poisoning) is relatively short and easily tracked. For example, if several people eat at a restaurant and then fall ill within a few days, it is easier to establish that the food exposure preceded the illness.

In contrast, **chronic diseases** like heart disease or cancer may take years or even decades to develop after the initial exposure. This makes establishing temporality more difficult, especially when exposures are intermittent or cumulative. In these cases, long-term cohort studies are essential for tracking exposures over time and determining whether those exposures truly precede the onset of disease.

For example, in studies of air pollution and chronic lung disease, it may take many years of monitoring both pollution levels and participants' health before researchers can conclude that exposure to pollutants was consistently higher before the development of lung disease.

Time Lag and Latency Period

Another important aspect of temporality is the concept of **latency period**—the time between exposure to a harmful agent and the appearance of the disease. For some diseases, the latency period is short. For others, like many cancers, the latency period can be decades. Understanding this time lag is critical in epidemiology because researchers need to follow participants long enough to detect any effects of the exposure.

For example, **mesothelioma**, a cancer caused by asbestos exposure, can take 20 to 50 years to develop after the initial exposure. In studies of asbestos workers, temporality is established only after following participants for a long time, during which cases of mesothelioma emerge among those exposed to asbestos years earlier.

Researchers also need to consider **cumulative exposure** over time. In conditions like cardiovascular disease, long-term exposure to risk factors like smoking or poor diet may have cumulative effects, where the total duration and intensity of exposure over many years is more important than short-term exposure.

Temporality in Public Health Interventions

In public health, understanding temporality is essential for designing interventions. If temporality is established, interventions can focus on **preventing exposure** before the disease develops. For example, knowing that smoking precedes lung cancer, public health campaigns aim to reduce smoking rates to prevent cancer years down the road. Similarly, by understanding that unprotected exposure to the sun occurs long before skin cancer develops, health officials can promote early interventions, such as the use of sunscreen in childhood to prevent skin cancer later in life.

Overall, establishing a **clear temporal sequence** is foundational for proving causality in epidemiological research. Without it, any association remains just that— an association—without evidence of a direct cause-and-effect relationship.

Dose-Response Relationships in Causal Analysis

A **dose-response relationship** refers to the correlation between the amount of exposure to a risk factor and the likelihood or severity of an outcome. When a higher level of exposure leads to an increased risk of disease, this provides strong evidence supporting a **causal relationship**. As mentioned, the presence of a dose-response relationship is one of the **Bradford Hill criteria** used to evaluate whether an observed association between exposure and outcome is likely to be causal.

Importance of Dose-Response Relationships

A dose-response relationship is important because it suggests that the exposure has a **biologically active role** in the development of the disease. If a small amount of an exposure causes mild harm and a larger amount causes greater harm, this stepwise increase strengthens the argument that the exposure is responsible for the outcome. For example, studies of smoking and lung cancer have shown that individuals who smoke more cigarettes per day or for a longer duration are at a greater risk of developing lung cancer. This graded relationship supports the idea that smoking is a causal factor in lung cancer development.

Quantifying exposure is key to studying dose-response relationships. Exposure can be measured in various ways, such as intensity (e.g., how many cigarettes a person smokes per day), duration (e.g., how many years they've smoked), or cumulative exposure (e.g., total number of cigarettes smoked over a lifetime). The stronger and more consistent the dose-response relationship, the more convincing the evidence that the exposure is contributing to the outcome.

Examples of Dose-Response Relationships

Smoking and lung cancer is one of the clearest examples of a dose-response relationship. Numerous studies have shown that individuals who smoke more frequently or for a longer period have a higher risk of developing lung cancer. For instance, heavy smokers (e.g., 40 cigarettes a day) are far more likely to develop lung cancer than light smokers (e.g., 5 cigarettes a day), and both are at higher risk than non-smokers. This gradient suggests that the carcinogenic compounds in tobacco smoke have a cumulative effect on lung tissue, making it more likely for mutations to occur with increased exposure.

Another example can be seen in **alcohol consumption and liver disease**. Studies show that individuals who drink alcohol excessively over time have a higher risk of developing liver cirrhosis compared to light or moderate drinkers. The more alcohol a person consumes on a regular basis, the greater the damage to the liver, demonstrating a clear dose-response relationship.

In the realm of **occupational health**, exposure to **asbestos** and the risk of developing mesothelioma follows a similar pattern. Workers who were heavily exposed to asbestos fibers over many years are far more likely to develop mesothelioma compared to those who had minimal exposure. This demonstrates how increasing levels of exposure contribute to a higher risk of disease.

Threshold and Saturation Effects

While dose-response relationships are common, they are not always **linear**. In some cases, a **threshold effect** may exist, where a certain level of exposure is required before the risk of disease increases. Below this threshold, exposure may not result in any measurable harm. For example, low levels of radiation exposure may not cause noticeable health effects, but once a certain dose is exceeded, the risk of cancer increases significantly.

Conversely, some dose-response relationships exhibit **saturation effects**, where the risk of disease increases with exposure up to a point, but then plateaus. This happens when the biological system responsible for processing or responding to the exposure becomes overwhelmed or reaches its capacity. For instance, increasing dietary sodium intake can raise blood pressure, but at extremely high levels, the effect may plateau because the body cannot raise blood pressure indefinitely without causing acute damage or other physiological changes.

Nonlinear Dose-Response Relationships

Not all dose-response relationships are linear. Some exposures may have a **U-shaped** or **J-shaped** relationship with the outcome, where both very low and very high levels of exposure are associated with higher risks, and moderate exposure is associated with the lowest risk. This has been observed with **alcohol consumption** and cardiovascular disease, where light to moderate alcohol consumption is associated with a lower risk of heart disease, while heavy drinking increases the risk. Understanding these nonlinear patterns is critical in interpreting dose-response relationships and designing appropriate interventions.

Application in Public Health and Policy

Identifying and understanding dose-response relationships helps inform public health guidelines and policies. For example, if a strong dose-response relationship is found between air pollution levels and respiratory disease, governments can set **exposure limits** to reduce the population's overall risk. Similarly, dose-response findings in **occupational safety** might lead to stricter regulations on chemical exposures in the workplace to prevent long-term harm.

CHAPTER 10: INFECTIOUS DISEASE EPIDEMIOLOGY

Transmission Dynamics of Infectious Diseases

The **transmission dynamics** of infectious diseases refer to how diseases spread through populations, influenced by the nature of the pathogen, host behavior, and environmental factors. Understanding these dynamics is key to controlling outbreaks and preventing widespread infections.

Modes of Transmission

Infectious diseases can spread through several **modes of transmission: direct contact, indirect contact, droplet transmission, airborne transmission**, and **vector-borne transmission**. Each mode involves different pathways and risks.

- **Direct contact transmission** occurs when an infected individual physically transfers the pathogen to another person. This can happen through skin contact, sexual contact, or blood exchange, as seen with HIV or hepatitis B.
- **Indirect contact transmission** involves an intermediate object or surface. Pathogens can linger on surfaces such as doorknobs or medical instruments, which become contaminated when touched by an infected person. If someone else touches the contaminated object and then their face or mouth, they might become infected. Diseases like norovirus spread easily this way.
- **Droplet transmission** occurs when respiratory droplets carrying infectious agents are expelled during coughing, sneezing, or talking. These droplets, heavy and short-lived, usually spread within a few meters, making diseases like influenza or COVID-19 transmissible in close contact situations.
- **Airborne transmission** involves smaller particles (aerosols) that can remain suspended in the air for longer periods and over greater distances. Diseases like tuberculosis and measles spread through airborne routes, making them highly contagious in enclosed spaces.
- **Vector-borne transmission** involves organisms like mosquitoes, ticks, or fleas that carry pathogens from one host to another. Malaria, transmitted by mosquitoes, is a well-known example of vector-borne disease.

Understanding the specific mode of transmission helps epidemiologists design targeted interventions, such as isolation for direct contact diseases or vector control for malaria.

Basic Reproduction Number (R0)

The **basic reproduction number (R0)** is a key concept in transmission dynamics. R0 represents the average number of secondary infections produced by a single infected individual in a fully susceptible population. If R0 is greater than 1, the disease can spread widely; if it's less than 1, the disease will likely fade out over time.

For example, **measles** has a high R0, often around 12 to 18, meaning one infected person can transmit the virus to 12-18 others in a fully susceptible population. In contrast, **influenza** typically has an R0 of around 1.3 to 1.8, making it less transmissible than measles but still capable of causing significant outbreaks, especially in populations with low immunity.

R0 is influenced by factors such as the infectious period, mode of transmission, and the contact rate between individuals. Reducing R0 is the goal of many public health interventions, including vaccination programs, social distancing, and quarantine measures. For example, during the COVID-19 pandemic, measures like mask-wearing and lockdowns aimed to reduce the virus's R0 below 1 to control its spread.

Incubation and Infectious Periods

The **incubation period** is the time between exposure to the pathogen and the appearance of symptoms. It varies greatly between diseases. For example, the incubation period for **influenza** is typically 1 to 4 days, while for **hepatitis B**, it can range from 6 weeks to 6 months. The longer the incubation period, the more challenging it is to identify and isolate infected individuals before they can spread the disease.

The **infectious period** is the time during which an infected person can transmit the disease to others. For some diseases, people are most infectious just before or during the early stages of symptoms. For example, individuals infected with **COVID-19** are often most contagious a day or two before symptoms appear. Others, like people infected with **HIV**, can transmit the virus for years without showing symptoms, complicating prevention efforts.

Herd Immunity

Herd immunity occurs when a sufficient proportion of a population becomes immune to a disease, either through vaccination or previous infection, reducing the likelihood of disease spread. When enough people are immune, the pathogen's transmission chain is broken, protecting even those who are not immune. The threshold for achieving herd immunity depends on the disease's R0. Diseases with higher R0 values, like measles, require a greater percentage of the population to be immune (often above 90%) to prevent outbreaks.

Vaccination programs aim to achieve herd immunity by immunizing large portions of the population, reducing the number of susceptible individuals. This approach has led to the near eradication of diseases like **smallpox** and the substantial reduction of others, such as **polio** and **measles**, in many parts of the world.

Superspreading Events

Not all individuals contribute equally to the spread of infectious diseases. **Superspreaders** are people who, often due to high contact rates or specific biological factors, transmit the pathogen to a disproportionately large number of individuals. For example, a single person infected with **SARS** in 2003 was found to have transmitted the virus to over 100 other people during their stay in a hospital.

Superspreading events can significantly alter the dynamics of an outbreak. They often occur in crowded settings, such as hospitals, social gatherings, or public transportation, where an infected individual has extensive contact with others. Identifying and preventing superspreading events is crucial for controlling outbreaks, as these events can accelerate transmission and lead to more widespread infections.

Contact Networks and Transmission

Contact patterns within a population are influential in transmission dynamics. Diseases spread more easily in dense, well-connected populations where individuals frequently interact, as seen in urban areas. Contact networks describe how individuals in a population interact and can be mapped to show how infections might spread. For example, diseases like **influenza** spread rapidly in schools or workplaces where people are in close proximity.

Heterogeneity in contact patterns also affects disease transmission. While some individuals have few contacts, others, like healthcare workers, may interact with many people and thus have a higher likelihood of transmitting disease. Understanding these patterns helps epidemiologists design interventions, such as targeted vaccinations for high-contact individuals or groups, to reduce the risk of widespread transmission.

Basic Reproductive Number (R0) and Herd Immunity

The **basic reproductive number (R0)** is a key concept in infectious disease epidemiology, used to describe the contagiousness of a disease. R0 represents the average number of secondary infections that a single infected individual will cause in a fully susceptible population. In simpler terms, it quantifies how easily a disease spreads from one person to others in a population with no prior immunity or interventions like vaccines or treatments in place.

For example, if R0 equals 2, it means that, on average, each infected person will transmit the disease to two others. If R0 is greater than 1, the disease can potentially spread and cause an outbreak. If R0 is less than 1, the disease will likely fizzle out because each infected person is infecting fewer than one person on average, meaning the spread is not sustainable.

R0 is not a fixed number for any disease. It can vary depending on factors such as population density, social behavior, the effectiveness of health interventions, and environmental conditions. For instance, **influenza** typically has an R0 between 1.3 and 1.8, but in crowded, poorly ventilated spaces, the R0 could be higher. In contrast, **measles** has a much higher R0, often ranging from 12 to 18, making it one of the most contagious diseases known.

Factors Affecting R0

Several factors influence R0, making it a complex measure:

1. **Infectious period**: The longer someone remains contagious, the more time they have to transmit the infection to others. Diseases with longer infectious periods, like **tuberculosis**, tend to have a higher potential for spread if left unchecked.
2. **Mode of transmission**: Diseases that spread through the air (like measles) or via close, frequent contact (like influenza) typically have higher R0 values. In contrast, diseases that require specific routes, such as bloodborne viruses like **HIV**, tend to have lower R0 values.
3. **Contact rates**: The frequency and nature of interactions between individuals influence how quickly a disease spreads. In densely populated urban areas, the R0 might be higher than in rural, less populated settings because people come into contact more often.
4. **Susceptibility of the population**: R0 assumes that everyone in the population is susceptible to the disease. In real-world scenarios, factors like immunity (from previous infections or vaccination), public health measures (like quarantine or social distancing), and personal behaviors (like mask-wearing) reduce R0.

Herd Immunity

Herd immunity occurs when a sufficient proportion of the population becomes immune to a disease, either through vaccination or previous infection, making it less likely that the disease will spread. Herd immunity protects not only those who are immune but also those who are not (such as newborns, the elderly, or individuals with weakened immune systems), as the disease has fewer potential hosts to infect.

The threshold for achieving herd immunity is directly related to R0. The higher the R0, the larger the proportion of the population that needs to be immune to prevent outbreaks. The formula to calculate the herd immunity threshold is:

$$\text{Herd immunity threshold} = 1 - (1/R0)$$

For example, if the R0 of a disease is 2, then the herd immunity threshold is $1 - (1/2) = 0.5$, meaning 50% of the population needs to be immune to prevent the spread. For a disease like measles, with an R0 of around 12, the threshold is much higher: $1 - (1/12) = 0.92$, or 92% of the population must be immune for herd immunity to be effective.

Achieving Herd Immunity Through Vaccination

Vaccination is the most effective way to achieve herd immunity without causing widespread illness and death. Vaccines work by stimulating the immune system to develop antibodies against a pathogen, providing immunity without the individual having to endure the disease.

For highly contagious diseases like measles, achieving herd immunity through natural infection would require that nearly 90-95% of the population become infected, which could lead to high levels of morbidity and mortality. Vaccination programs, such as those for measles, polio, and diphtheria, have successfully reduced or eliminated outbreaks in many parts of the world by achieving the herd immunity threshold through immunization.

Herd Immunity and Public Health Policy

Herd immunity thresholds guide public health strategies. For example, during the COVID-19 pandemic, countries implemented mass vaccination campaigns to reduce the spread of the virus and lower its R0. However, achieving herd immunity is not always straightforward. Factors like **vaccine hesitancy**, **mutating pathogens**, and **unequal access to vaccines** can hinder efforts to reach the necessary level of immunity.

Mutations that make a pathogen more contagious can also raise the R0, thus raising the herd immunity threshold. For example, new variants of **SARS-CoV-2** with higher transmissibility require even more people to be vaccinated to control the spread, illustrating the dynamic nature of herd immunity thresholds.

In some cases, herd immunity can be regional. If vaccination coverage is high in one country but low in another, outbreaks can still occur in under-vaccinated areas, even if the overall global population is closer to herd immunity. This highlights the importance of global vaccination efforts, especially in interconnected societies.

Epidemic and Endemic Patterns

Infectious diseases can manifest in different patterns within populations, commonly described as **epidemic**, **endemic**, or **pandemic**. Understanding these patterns helps epidemiologists track diseases and design appropriate interventions.

Epidemic Patterns

An **epidemic** occurs when there is a sudden increase in the number of cases of a disease above what is normally expected in a specific population or area. Epidemics are often triggered by a change in the infectious agent, a new susceptible population, or environmental factors that facilitate disease spread. For instance, the 2014-2016 **Ebola epidemic** in West Africa saw a dramatic rise in cases due to a combination of poor healthcare infrastructure, high transmission rates, and delayed response efforts.

Epidemics can be local, affecting just one community, or they can spread across larger regions, as seen with **seasonal influenza** outbreaks. Epidemics usually exhibit a **sharp increase** in cases, a peak, and then a decline as the population either gains immunity or effective public health interventions are implemented. **Point-source epidemics**, like a foodborne outbreak, often have a sharp, short-lived spike in cases, whereas **propagated epidemics**, like measles, can show more sustained transmission as the disease spreads from person to person over time.

The factors that lead to epidemics include:

1. **Introduction of a new pathogen** into a population with no prior immunity (e.g., the emergence of **HIV** in the 1980s).
2. **Changes in the pathogen**, such as mutations that increase its transmissibility or evade immunity, seen with **SARS-CoV-2** variants.
3. **Increased susceptibility** in the population, often due to a decline in vaccination rates, such as the resurgence of **measles** in areas where vaccination coverage dropped.
4. **Environmental or social changes**, such as natural disasters, wars, or mass gatherings, which facilitate transmission.

Endemic Patterns

In contrast, an **endemic** disease is one that is consistently present within a population or geographic area, but the number of cases remains relatively stable over time. Endemic diseases occur at predictable rates and are considered the "normal" baseline for that disease in a specific region. For example, **malaria** is endemic in many tropical regions, where it persists at relatively steady levels due to the presence of the **Anopheles mosquito**, the disease's vector, and environmental conditions that support transmission.

Endemicity reflects a balance between transmission and immunity in the population. For a disease to remain endemic, enough people must remain susceptible over time for the pathogen to continue circulating. This can happen through new births (adding susceptible individuals), waning immunity, or incomplete vaccination coverage. Diseases like **tuberculosis** remain endemic in certain regions, especially where social and environmental conditions—such as overcrowding or poverty—allow ongoing transmission.

Transition Between Epidemic and Endemic

A disease can transition between epidemic and endemic states based on changes in population immunity or interventions. For example, **dengue fever** often fluctuates between epidemic outbreaks and endemic circulation in tropical regions. After a large epidemic, immunity within the population may rise temporarily, reducing transmission until immunity wanes or new susceptible individuals enter the population, allowing for another outbreak.

Public health efforts, such as widespread vaccination, can help shift a disease from epidemic to endemic or even eradicate it. **Smallpox**, once a global epidemic threat, was eradicated through a concerted vaccination campaign that interrupted transmission worldwide.

Pandemic Patterns

A **pandemic** is a global epidemic, where the disease spreads across multiple countries and affects a large number of people. Pandemics occur when a new infectious agent emerges, with little to no pre-existing immunity in the global population. The **COVID-19 pandemic** is a prime example, where the novel coronavirus rapidly spread across the world due to its high transmissibility and the lack of prior immunity.

Pandemics often start as local epidemics before spreading widely. The 1918 influenza pandemic, for instance, began as localized outbreaks but quickly spread across the globe due to the high mobility of people during and after World War I. Pandemics typically result in more severe public health crises because the spread is widespread, overwhelming healthcare systems, and requiring international cooperation to control.

Pandemics differ from epidemics primarily in **scale and geographic spread**. While an epidemic may be confined to a single country or region, a pandemic affects multiple countries or continents. The **COVID-19 pandemic** is a clear example of how a localized epidemic in one region (Wuhan, China) can quickly escalate into a pandemic due to the rapid global movement of people and the interconnectedness of modern societies.

Public Health Implications

Both **epidemic** and **endemic** patterns have important public health implications. During epidemics, public health officials must act quickly to implement **surveillance**, **contact tracing**, **quarantines**, and **vaccination campaigns** to prevent further spread. In the case of endemic diseases, the focus is often on **long-term control strategies**, such as regular immunization programs, vector control in the case of diseases like malaria, and improving healthcare access to manage ongoing disease transmission.

For **epidemics**, the goal is often to stop the spread before it becomes widespread, whereas for **endemic diseases**, the objective is to keep disease rates as low and stable as possible. Public health resources are allocated accordingly. During an epidemic, surge capacity—such as setting up temporary hospitals or increasing diagnostic testing—is critical, while for endemic diseases, the emphasis is on sustaining healthcare infrastructure over time.

Shifting Patterns and Emerging Threats

Infectious diseases can shift between epidemic and endemic patterns due to several factors, including **climate change**, **urbanization**, **global travel**, and **changes in population immunity**. For example, diseases like **dengue fever**, historically endemic to tropical regions, have started appearing in regions outside the tropics due to changes in global temperatures and the spread of the mosquito vector.

Moreover, **antimicrobial resistance** (AMR) poses a significant threat to controlling both epidemic and endemic diseases. As bacteria, viruses, and other pathogens develop resistance to current treatments, diseases that were once manageable can become harder to control, potentially leading to more frequent and severe outbreaks.

CHAPTER 11: CHRONIC DISEASE EPIDEMIOLOGY

Common Chronic Diseases (Cardiovascular, Cancer, Diabetes)

Chronic diseases are long-term health conditions that progress slowly and persist over time, often leading to disability or death if unmanaged. Three of the most common and burdensome chronic diseases are **cardiovascular disease**, **cancer**, and **diabetes**. These conditions not only cause significant morbidity and mortality but also create substantial healthcare costs and strain on public health systems.

Cardiovascular Disease

Cardiovascular disease (CVD) refers to a group of disorders that affect the heart and blood vessels, with **coronary artery disease (CAD)** and **stroke** being the most common forms. CAD occurs when the coronary arteries become narrowed or blocked due to the buildup of plaque, reducing blood flow to the heart muscle. This can lead to **angina** (chest pain) or a **myocardial infarction** (heart attack). **Stroke** results from interrupted blood supply to the brain, either due to a clot (ischemic stroke) or a burst blood vessel (hemorrhagic stroke).

Several risk factors increase the likelihood of developing CVD, including **hypertension** (high blood pressure), **high cholesterol levels, smoking, physical inactivity**, and **unhealthy diets. Obesity** and **diabetes** are also major contributors. Studies show that hypertension alone is responsible for a significant proportion of strokes and heart attacks globally, making it a primary target for intervention.

The **epidemiology** of cardiovascular disease has shifted in recent decades. While rates of CVD have declined in many high-income countries due to improved medical care and lifestyle changes, they continue to rise in low- and middle-income nations where lifestyle changes like urbanization and diets high in processed foods are becoming more common. This shifting burden highlights the importance of prevention efforts targeting **modifiable risk factors** like diet, exercise, and smoking cessation.

Cancer

Cancer is characterized by the uncontrolled growth of abnormal cells in the body. It can develop in almost any organ and spread to other parts of the body (metastasis). The most common types of cancer globally are **lung, breast, colorectal**, and **prostate cancer**, though many other forms exist. The burden of cancer is growing worldwide, with millions of new cases diagnosed each year.

Cancer develops due to genetic mutations, which can be influenced by environmental exposures, lifestyle factors, and inherited genetic predispositions. **Tobacco use** is the leading preventable cause of cancer, responsible for around 22% of global cancer deaths, particularly **lung cancer**. In addition to smoking, **alcohol consumption**, **exposure to carcinogens** like asbestos and UV radiation, **poor diet**, and **lack of physical activity** increase the risk of various cancers. Certain **infections**, such as **human papillomavirus (HPV)** and **hepatitis B**, are also linked to cancers like **cervical** and **liver cancer**, respectively.

Cancer epidemiology focuses on identifying risk factors and understanding how they contribute to different cancer types. Screening programs for cancers like **breast**, **cervical**, and **colorectal cancer** have proven effective in reducing mortality by detecting disease at earlier, more treatable stages. However, disparities in access to screening and treatment mean that outcomes vary significantly across populations. For instance, in high-income countries, cancer survival rates are generally higher due to early detection and access to advanced treatments. In low-income regions, limited healthcare access results in later diagnoses and higher mortality rates.

Preventive measures like smoking cessation, vaccination (e.g., for HPV), and reducing occupational exposures to carcinogens are essential for lowering cancer incidence. In addition, **public health campaigns** that promote healthy diets, physical activity, and regular screening can reduce the cancer burden across populations.

Diabetes

Diabetes is a chronic condition characterized by the body's inability to properly regulate blood glucose levels. The two primary types are **Type 1 diabetes**, an autoimmune condition where the body attacks insulin-producing cells, and **Type 2 diabetes**, which results from the body's resistance to insulin or inadequate insulin production. Type 2 diabetes accounts for over 90% of all diabetes cases worldwide and is closely linked to **obesity**, **physical inactivity**, and **poor dietary habits**.

Diabetes significantly increases the risk of developing cardiovascular diseases, **kidney failure**, **blindness**, and **amputations** due to its impact on the body's organs and circulation. Uncontrolled diabetes leads to **hyperglycemia**, where elevated blood sugar levels damage tissues over time, contributing to these severe complications. In addition, diabetes often coexists with other conditions, such as hypertension and high cholesterol, which further elevate health risks.

The global prevalence of diabetes has risen dramatically in recent decades, particularly in low- and middle-income countries where rapid urbanization, changes in diet, and sedentary lifestyles are becoming more common. The **epidemiology of diabetes** reveals significant geographic and demographic disparities. For example, diabetes prevalence is particularly high in regions like South Asia, the

Middle East, and parts of the Pacific Islands, where genetic predisposition combined with changing lifestyles has fueled the epidemic.

Prevention of Type 2 diabetes focuses heavily on lifestyle interventions, including weight management, healthy eating, and regular physical activity. Population-wide strategies that promote access to healthy foods, create environments that encourage physical activity, and provide education on managing risk factors can prevent or delay the onset of diabetes. Additionally, early detection through screening and management with **medications** like **metformin** can prevent complications and improve quality of life for those living with diabetes.

Risk Factors for Chronic Diseases

Chronic diseases, such as cardiovascular disease, cancer, and diabetes, share a set of **modifiable and non-modifiable risk factors** that contribute to their development. Understanding these risk factors helps guide preventive measures and public health strategies aimed at reducing the global burden of these conditions.

1. Modifiable Risk Factors

Modifiable risk factors are those that individuals can change or manage through lifestyle adjustments or interventions. These include behaviors, environmental exposures, and physiological conditions that can be influenced by public health programs and individual actions.

- **Tobacco Use:** Smoking is one of the leading risk factors for many chronic diseases, particularly **lung cancer, cardiovascular disease**, and **chronic obstructive pulmonary disease (COPD)**. It contributes to about 22% of global cancer deaths and is responsible for a significant proportion of deaths from heart disease and stroke. Smoking cessation is one of the most effective ways to reduce the risk of these chronic conditions.
- **Unhealthy Diet:** Diets high in **saturated fats, trans fats, sugar**, and **salt** increase the risk of developing **obesity, type 2 diabetes, hypertension**, and **heart disease**. In particular, diets rich in **processed foods**, sugary beverages, and red or processed meats have been linked to higher rates of chronic diseases like colorectal cancer and cardiovascular disease. **Inadequate intake of fruits and vegetables** is another dietary factor contributing to these diseases.
- **Physical Inactivity:** A sedentary lifestyle significantly increases the risk of **obesity, type 2 diabetes, heart disease**, and certain cancers, such as breast and colon cancer. Regular physical activity, including moderate-intensity exercises like walking or cycling, helps maintain a healthy weight, regulate blood sugar, and lower blood pressure, reducing the risk of chronic diseases.

- **Alcohol Consumption**: Excessive alcohol consumption is linked to several chronic conditions, including **liver cirrhosis**, **cancer** (particularly of the liver, breast, and mouth), and **hypertension**. While moderate alcohol consumption may have some protective effects against heart disease, excessive drinking poses significant health risks.
- **Obesity**: Obesity is a major risk factor for many chronic diseases, including **type 2 diabetes**, **heart disease**, **stroke**, and several types of cancer (such as breast, colorectal, and pancreatic cancers). It is closely tied to poor diet and physical inactivity, and it exacerbates other risk factors like high cholesterol and hypertension.
- **Environmental Exposures**: Exposure to **pollution, occupational hazards**, and **carcinogens** such as **asbestos, pesticides**, and **airborne particulates** increases the risk of various chronic diseases. Air pollution, in particular, is a significant risk factor for **respiratory diseases** and **cardiovascular conditions**.

2. Non-Modifiable Risk Factors

Non-modifiable risk factors are those beyond an individual's control, such as **genetics**, **age**, and **gender**. These factors can still have a major role in chronic disease development.

- **Age**: The risk of developing most chronic diseases increases with age. For instance, **cardiovascular disease**, **cancer**, and **type 2 diabetes** are more common in older populations. As life expectancy increases worldwide, more people are living longer with chronic diseases.
- **Genetics and Family History**: A person's genetic makeup can predispose them to certain chronic diseases. For example, a family history of **heart disease**, **breast cancer**, or **diabetes** increases an individual's risk of developing these conditions. Specific genetic mutations, like the **BRCA1 and BRCA2** mutations, are strongly associated with increased risk for **breast** and **ovarian cancers**.
- **Ethnicity**: Certain ethnic groups have higher risks for specific chronic diseases due to a combination of genetic, environmental, and socio-economic factors. For example, people of **South Asian** descent are more likely to develop **type 2 diabetes** at a lower body mass index (BMI) compared to other groups. Similarly, **African Americans** are more likely to suffer from **hypertension** and its complications, such as stroke.
- **Gender**: Men and women can have different risks for chronic diseases. For instance, **cardiovascular disease** tends to develop earlier in men but becomes a significant risk for women after menopause. On the other hand, women are more likely to develop certain cancers, like **breast cancer**, and conditions like **osteoporosis** as they age.

3. Socioeconomic and Psychological Factors

Socioeconomic factors, such as income, education, and access to healthcare, also influence chronic disease risk. Individuals from lower socioeconomic backgrounds often face higher risks due to limited access to healthcare, healthier food options, and opportunities for physical activity. **Chronic stress** and **mental health conditions** like **depression** are also associated with an increased risk of chronic diseases. Long-term stress can contribute to **hypertension**, **heart disease**, and **type 2 diabetes**, partly through its effects on behavior, such as overeating, smoking, or physical inactivity.

Challenges in Chronic Disease Prevention and Control

Preventing and controlling chronic diseases presents several **public health challenges**, despite the fact that many of these diseases are preventable through lifestyle changes and medical interventions.

1. Lifestyle and Behavior Change

One of the main challenges in preventing chronic diseases is encouraging and sustaining **behavioral changes**. Habits like **smoking**, **poor diet**, and **physical inactivity** are deeply ingrained in daily life and influenced by numerous external factors, such as environment, culture, and socioeconomic status. Convincing individuals to adopt healthier behaviors is difficult because lifestyle changes often require long-term commitment and may conflict with societal norms or personal preferences. For example, many people may not have access to affordable, healthy food or safe places to exercise, making it harder to maintain healthier behaviors.

Public health campaigns that promote awareness are essential, but they are often insufficient by themselves. Effective interventions require multifaceted approaches that include **education**, **community-based initiatives**, and **policies** that make healthier choices easier. For example, taxing sugary drinks, promoting **smoke-free environments**, or creating **bike-friendly cities** can support individual efforts to adopt healthier behaviors.

2. Health Inequities

There are significant **disparities** in chronic disease prevention and care based on **socioeconomic status**, **race**, **ethnicity**, and **geographic location**. Individuals from lower-income communities or marginalized groups often face higher rates of chronic diseases due to reduced access to healthcare, healthy food, and preventive services. Addressing these inequities is a major public health challenge. Improving access to quality healthcare and preventive services for these populations is crucial but often requires systemic changes, such as increasing healthcare funding, expanding insurance coverage, and addressing **social determinants of health** like housing and education.

3. Healthcare System Limitations

Chronic diseases require long-term management and care, placing a significant burden on healthcare systems. Many healthcare models are designed to address

acute illnesses rather than providing continuous care for **chronic conditions**. This leads to gaps in care, especially for individuals with multiple chronic diseases who require **multidisciplinary** approaches. Coordinating care between primary care providers, specialists, and other healthcare professionals can be difficult, and fragmented care often leads to poor disease management.

Furthermore, healthcare systems are often more reactive than preventive, meaning resources are directed at treating diseases after they develop rather than investing in preventive measures. Shifting resources toward **prevention**, such as screening programs and early interventions, could significantly reduce the overall burden of chronic diseases, but this requires both political will and upfront investment.

4. Globalization and Urbanization

Rapid **urbanization** and **globalization** contribute to the spread of unhealthy behaviors, such as increased consumption of processed foods, sedentary lifestyles, and smoking. In many low- and middle-income countries, the transition from traditional diets and active lifestyles to more Westernized patterns has led to rising rates of chronic diseases. Urbanization also increases exposure to environmental risk factors like **air pollution**, which is associated with diseases like **cardiovascular disease** and **lung cancer**. Tackling these issues on a global scale requires international cooperation and coordinated public health policies that address these emerging challenges.

In short, chronic disease prevention and control require addressing complex challenges at both the individual and systemic levels. Promoting sustained lifestyle changes, reducing health disparities, strengthening healthcare systems, and managing the effects of urbanization and globalization are all essential steps in reducing the growing burden of chronic diseases.

CHAPTER 12: ENVIRONMENTAL AND OCCUPATIONAL EPIDEMIOLOGY

Impact of Environmental Exposures on Health

Environmental exposures have a profound impact on human health, influencing the development of various diseases and health conditions. These exposures come from a wide range of sources, including air and water pollution, hazardous chemicals, radiation, and climate-related factors. Understanding how these environmental factors affect health is critical for developing public health policies and interventions aimed at reducing harmful exposures.

Air Pollution and Respiratory Health

Air pollution is one of the most significant environmental exposures that impacts health, particularly **respiratory and cardiovascular diseases**. Pollutants such as **particulate matter (PM2.5), nitrogen dioxide (NO2)**, and **ozone (O3)** are released from industrial activities, vehicle emissions, and burning of fossil fuels. These pollutants are inhaled into the lungs, where they cause inflammation and damage to respiratory tissues. Long-term exposure to air pollution is strongly linked to **chronic obstructive pulmonary disease (COPD), asthma**, and **lung cancer**.

Children and the elderly are especially vulnerable to the effects of air pollution. In children, early exposure to high levels of air pollution can stunt lung development, increasing the risk of respiratory problems later in life. Studies have also shown that people living in areas with high pollution levels experience higher rates of **hospitalizations** for asthma and other respiratory conditions.

The **cardiovascular system** is also affected by air pollution. Fine particulate matter can enter the bloodstream and cause systemic inflammation, leading to **atherosclerosis** and increased risk of **heart attacks** and **stroke**. Research shows that even short-term spikes in air pollution levels can trigger cardiovascular events, especially in individuals with pre-existing heart conditions.

Water Pollution and Health Outcomes

Contaminated water sources pose serious health risks, particularly in low- and middle-income countries where access to clean water may be limited. **Water pollution** can result from agricultural runoff, industrial waste, and inadequate wastewater treatment, introducing harmful chemicals and pathogens into drinking water supplies. **Heavy metals** such as **lead, arsenic**, and **mercury** are common water contaminants that have been linked to a variety of health problems.

Lead exposure, for example, can result in **neurodevelopmental issues** in children, affecting their cognitive abilities and behavior. Long-term exposure to lead in drinking water, often from corroding pipes, can lead to permanent damage to the brain and nervous system. Arsenic, another toxic contaminant, is associated with **skin lesions**, **cardiovascular disease**, and **cancer**—particularly of the bladder, lungs, and skin.

In addition to chemical contaminants, **microbial pollution** in water supplies causes diseases such as **cholera**, **dysentery**, and **typhoid fever**. In areas without proper sanitation, contaminated water leads to outbreaks of diarrheal diseases, which are a leading cause of mortality among children under five years old globally.

Chemical Exposures and Cancer Risk

Exposure to **hazardous chemicals** in the environment has been linked to the development of several cancers. **Carcinogens** such as **asbestos**, **benzene**, and **pesticides** increase cancer risk by damaging DNA and promoting abnormal cell growth.

For example, **asbestos**, which was widely used in construction materials, is a known cause of **mesothelioma**, a rare but aggressive cancer that affects the lining of the lungs. Occupational exposure to asbestos, especially among construction workers and miners, has been strongly associated with this type of cancer, even decades after the initial exposure.

Pesticides used in agriculture have also been linked to cancers such as **non-Hodgkin lymphoma** and **leukemia**. Farmers and agricultural workers who handle these chemicals are at higher risk due to prolonged exposure. In communities near agricultural areas, **pesticide drift**—where chemicals sprayed on crops are carried by the wind—can also lead to increased cancer risk among residents.

Climate Change and Health Impacts

The growing impact of **climate change** is also influencing patterns of disease and exposure to environmental hazards. Rising global temperatures contribute to the spread of **vector-borne diseases** like **malaria** and **dengue fever**, as warmer climates expand the habitats of mosquitoes and other vectors. This means that diseases that were once confined to tropical regions are now appearing in more temperate zones, putting new populations at risk.

Extreme weather events, such as **heatwaves**, **floods**, and **hurricanes**, are becoming more frequent due to climate change, posing additional health risks. Heatwaves are associated with increased mortality from **heatstroke** and exacerbate conditions like heart disease and respiratory illness. **Flooding** increases the risk of waterborne diseases and can lead to contamination of drinking water supplies, further increasing health risks.

Indoor Environmental Exposures

Indoor environments can also be sources of harmful exposures. **Indoor air pollution**, caused by **tobacco smoke, mold, radon,** and **household chemicals**, contributes to respiratory diseases and cancer. In low-income countries, the use of **biomass fuels** for cooking and heating in poorly ventilated homes leads to high levels of indoor air pollution, resulting in respiratory illnesses, particularly among women and children who spend more time indoors.

Radon, a naturally occurring radioactive gas that can seep into homes from the soil, is the second leading cause of lung cancer after smoking. High radon levels in poorly ventilated basements and ground floors can expose occupants to this invisible hazard without their knowledge.

Occupational Hazards and Related Diseases

Occupational hazards are exposures or conditions in the workplace that pose risks to the health and safety of workers. These hazards vary across industries, but they often lead to specific diseases or injuries based on the nature of the work environment. Understanding these hazards is essential for preventing work-related illnesses and improving workplace safety.

1. Physical Hazards

Physical hazards include factors like noise, vibration, extreme temperatures, and radiation. Long-term exposure to high levels of noise, such as in manufacturing or construction, can lead to **noise-induced hearing loss**. Workers in these industries may not notice the gradual damage until significant hearing loss has occurred.

Exposure to **vibration**, often in jobs involving heavy machinery or power tools, can result in **hand-arm vibration syndrome (HAVS)**. This condition affects circulation and nerves in the hands, leading to symptoms such as numbness, tingling, and reduced grip strength.

Extreme temperatures also pose significant risks. In outdoor work environments or industrial settings, workers exposed to high heat may suffer from **heat-related illnesses** like **heat exhaustion** or **heat stroke**. Cold environments can lead to **frostbite** and **hypothermia**, especially in jobs that require long hours in freezing conditions, such as construction work in colder climates.

2. Chemical Hazards

Chemical hazards in the workplace arise from exposure to toxic substances, including gases, solvents, pesticides, and heavy metals. Workers in industries such as agriculture, manufacturing, and mining are at higher risk of coming into contact with harmful chemicals.

Exposure to **asbestos**, a material used in construction and insulation, can lead to **mesothelioma**, a rare but aggressive cancer of the lung lining. Asbestos exposure is also linked to **asbestosis** and **lung cancer**, with symptoms sometimes not appearing until decades after exposure.

In **agriculture**, workers exposed to **pesticides** may develop conditions like **pesticide poisoning**, which causes symptoms ranging from headaches and dizziness to more severe outcomes like neurological damage. Prolonged exposure to certain pesticides has also been linked to **non-Hodgkin lymphoma** and other cancers.

Heavy metals such as **lead** and **mercury** are another common occupational hazard. Workers exposed to lead in industries like battery manufacturing or construction may suffer from **lead poisoning**, which can affect the nervous system and cause cognitive impairments, especially in younger workers. Mercury exposure, common in industries like mining and electronics, can lead to **mercury poisoning**, causing neurological and kidney damage.

3. Biological Hazards

Occupational exposure to **biological hazards**, such as bacteria, viruses, and fungi, is particularly prevalent in healthcare settings, agriculture, and laboratories. **Healthcare workers** face a heightened risk of contracting **bloodborne diseases**, such as **hepatitis B**, **hepatitis C**, and **HIV**, through needlestick injuries or contact with infected bodily fluids.

In agriculture, workers can contract diseases like **zoonoses**—infections that spread from animals to humans. For example, **brucellosis** and **anthrax** can be contracted from livestock, while **avian influenza** may be transmitted from birds.

4. Ergonomic Hazards

Ergonomic hazards relate to how work is physically structured and performed. Jobs that require repetitive movements, poor posture, or heavy lifting can lead to **musculoskeletal disorders (MSDs)**. Common conditions include **carpal tunnel syndrome**, **tendinitis**, and **lower back pain**. Workers in jobs like assembly line work, warehouse jobs, and office work where repetitive strain is common are particularly at risk. Long hours spent sitting or performing repetitive tasks can exacerbate these conditions, leading to chronic pain and disability.

5. Psychosocial Hazards

Psychosocial hazards include workplace stress, harassment, and burnout. High-pressure work environments, long hours, and lack of job control contribute to mental health issues such as **depression, anxiety**, and **burnout**. Chronic stress from demanding jobs, particularly in professions like teaching, healthcare, and emergency services, is associated with an increased risk of **cardiovascular diseases**

and **sleep disorders**. Workplace bullying and harassment can also exacerbate mental health issues, leading to absenteeism and decreased job satisfaction.

The Role of Air, Water, and Chemical Pollutants in Disease

Environmental pollutants—whether found in the air, water, or soil—are significant contributors to a range of diseases. These pollutants stem from industrial activities, transportation, agriculture, and urbanization, exposing people to harmful chemicals and compounds that impact their health over time.

1. Air Pollutants

Air pollution is one of the most studied environmental risk factors for disease. Common air pollutants include **particulate matter (PM2.5 and PM10), nitrogen oxides (NOx), sulfur dioxide (SO2)**, and **volatile organic compounds (VOCs)**, all of which have detrimental health effects.

Particulate matter (PM), especially PM2.5, is made up of tiny particles that can penetrate deep into the lungs, causing **respiratory diseases** such as **asthma, bronchitis**, and **chronic obstructive pulmonary disease (COPD)**. Long-term exposure to particulate matter is also linked to **lung cancer**. Additionally, fine particles can enter the bloodstream, contributing to **cardiovascular diseases**, including heart attacks and strokes.

Ozone (O3), another significant pollutant, irritates the respiratory system, particularly in children, the elderly, and individuals with pre-existing conditions like asthma. Prolonged exposure can lead to the worsening of chronic lung diseases and increase the risk of premature death from respiratory causes.

2. Water Pollutants

Contaminated water supplies, particularly in regions with inadequate water treatment facilities, expose populations to both **chemical** and **microbial pollutants**. Heavy metals, such as **lead, arsenic**, and **mercury**, are commonly found in polluted water and have significant health consequences.

Lead, often from corroding pipes or industrial waste, causes **neurological damage**, particularly in children. Even low levels of lead exposure can affect cognitive development, leading to learning disabilities and behavioral problems. In adults, long-term exposure to lead can lead to **hypertension** and **kidney damage**.

Arsenic in drinking water, particularly in parts of South Asia, is a major public health issue. Chronic exposure to arsenic is linked to **skin lesions, bladder cancer**, and **cardiovascular disease**. Ingesting arsenic-contaminated water over long periods is also associated with **diabetes** and adverse birth outcomes.

Waterborne pathogens such as **E. coli, Salmonella,** and **Vibrio cholerae** cause diseases like **cholera** and **dysentery**, particularly in areas with poor sanitation. These infections lead to diarrheal diseases, which are a leading cause of death among children in developing countries.

3. Chemical Pollutants

Chemical pollutants, especially from industrial and agricultural activities, contribute to a range of chronic diseases. **Pesticides,** for example, are commonly used in farming but pose significant health risks to both workers and nearby populations. **Long-term exposure** to certain pesticides has been linked to cancers such as **leukemia** and **non-Hodgkin lymphoma**. Farmworkers who handle these chemicals are at particularly high risk, but pesticide drift can affect surrounding communities as well.

Polychlorinated biphenyls (PCBs) and **dioxins,** by-products of industrial processes, persist in the environment and accumulate in the food chain. These chemicals are classified as **endocrine disruptors,** interfering with hormonal systems and increasing the risk of cancers, **thyroid disorders,** and **reproductive health issues**.

In urban areas, exposure to **benzene,** a component of car exhaust and industrial emissions, is linked to **leukemia** and other blood disorders. Chronic exposure, even at low levels, poses significant risks to human health.

Climate-Related Health Risks and Emerging Environmental Hazards

As the global climate changes, new health risks and environmental hazards are emerging, posing significant challenges for public health systems worldwide. Rising temperatures, shifting weather patterns, and extreme weather events are directly and indirectly affecting human health. These climate-related changes exacerbate existing environmental hazards while introducing new ones, making it essential to understand and address the evolving risks.

Heat-Related Illnesses

One of the most immediate and direct health effects of climate change is **heat-related illnesses**. As global temperatures rise, the frequency and intensity of **heatwaves** are increasing, placing vulnerable populations such as the elderly, children, and people with pre-existing health conditions at higher risk. Heatwaves can cause **heat exhaustion, heatstroke,** and even **death,** particularly in regions unaccustomed to extreme heat. Prolonged exposure to high temperatures also exacerbates chronic conditions like **cardiovascular** and **respiratory diseases,** as the body struggles to regulate its internal temperature.

Urban areas are particularly vulnerable to heat-related risks due to the **urban heat island effect**, where concrete and asphalt trap heat, making cities significantly warmer than surrounding rural areas. This can lead to higher rates of heat-related hospital admissions and deaths in cities during heatwaves.

Air Quality and Respiratory Diseases

Climate change is also worsening **air quality**, contributing to respiratory diseases. Higher temperatures increase the formation of **ground-level ozone (O3)**, a harmful air pollutant that exacerbates **asthma** and other respiratory conditions. Additionally, changes in climate are lengthening the **pollen season**, leading to increased cases of **allergic reactions** and **asthma** flare-ups. The combination of higher temperatures, prolonged pollen seasons, and increased ozone levels places a greater burden on individuals with pre-existing respiratory conditions.

Moreover, **wildfires**—which are becoming more frequent and intense due to drier and hotter conditions—release large amounts of **particulate matter (PM2.5)** and other pollutants into the air. Wildfire smoke is highly toxic and can travel long distances, affecting the respiratory health of populations far from the fire's source. Inhaling smoke from wildfires is linked to worsening asthma, bronchitis, and long-term lung damage.

Waterborne and Vector-Borne Diseases

Shifting climate patterns are altering the distribution of **waterborne** and **vector-borne diseases**, creating new risks for populations that were previously unaffected.

Changes in rainfall patterns and flooding are increasing the spread of **waterborne diseases** such as **cholera**, **dysentery**, and **leptospirosis**. In regions with inadequate sanitation and water infrastructure, flooding can contaminate drinking water supplies with pathogens, leading to outbreaks of diarrheal diseases. Warmer temperatures also promote the growth of harmful bacteria and algae in water systems, increasing the risk of exposure to waterborne pathogens.

Climate change is also expanding the geographical range of **vector-borne diseases**. As temperatures rise, insects like **mosquitoes** and **ticks** can survive in previously inhospitable areas, bringing diseases such as **malaria, dengue fever, Zika virus**, and **Lyme disease** to new regions. For example, **malaria**, once confined to tropical and subtropical regions, is now spreading to higher altitudes and more temperate zones as mosquitoes thrive in warmer climates. This shift puts previously unaffected populations at risk and requires changes in public health surveillance and control strategies.

Food Security and Malnutrition

Climate change is affecting **agricultural productivity** and food security, which can lead to malnutrition and food-related health problems. Droughts, extreme weather events, and shifting growing seasons are reducing crop yields, leading to food shortages and higher prices. This can result in malnutrition, especially in low-income communities that rely on agriculture for both food and income.

Malnutrition weakens the immune system, making people more vulnerable to infectious diseases. Additionally, changing climate conditions can impact the **nutritional quality** of crops. Studies have shown that elevated carbon dioxide levels can reduce the concentrations of essential nutrients such as **protein, iron,** and **zinc** in staple crops like wheat and rice, further exacerbating malnutrition.

Mental Health and Climate Anxiety

The psychological impacts of climate change are often overlooked but are increasingly recognized as a significant health concern. **Mental health issues** such as **anxiety, depression,** and **post-traumatic stress disorder (PTSD)** are becoming more common as people experience the effects of climate-related disasters such as hurricanes, floods, and wildfires. The destruction of homes, displacement, and loss of livelihoods contribute to stress and anxiety, while the uncertainty of future climate risks creates **climate anxiety**, particularly among younger populations.

Emerging Environmental Hazards

In addition to the direct impacts of climate change, new **environmental hazards** are emerging. **Permafrost thawing** in the Arctic, for instance, could release **long-dormant pathogens** and **greenhouse gases** such as methane, potentially triggering new infectious diseases and accelerating global warming. Melting ice sheets also contribute to rising sea levels, increasing the risk of **coastal flooding** and **saltwater intrusion** into freshwater systems, which can affect drinking water supplies and agricultural land.

Furthermore, climate change is influencing **chemical exposure** risks. Higher temperatures can increase the volatility and spread of certain pollutants, such as pesticides and industrial chemicals, while extreme weather events can damage infrastructure and release hazardous materials into the environment, posing risks to both human health and ecosystems.

CHAPTER 13: SOCIAL DETERMINANTS OF HEALTH IN EPIDEMIOLOGY

Socioeconomic Status and Health Disparities

In epidemiology, **socioeconomic status (SES)** is one of the most powerful predictors of health outcomes. SES refers to an individual or group's economic and social standing, typically measured by income, education level, and occupation. These factors influence a person's access to resources, opportunities, and environments that shape health. Lower SES is consistently linked to poorer health outcomes, while higher SES generally correlates with better health.

Income and Health

Income is a fundamental aspect of socioeconomic status, affecting nearly every dimension of health. People with higher incomes can afford better housing, healthier food, quality healthcare, and access to preventive services. In contrast, those with lower incomes often face limited choices in these areas, leading to poorer health.

For example, low-income individuals may live in neighborhoods with higher pollution levels, less access to safe recreational areas, and fewer grocery stores offering fresh produce. These environmental constraints increase the likelihood of developing **chronic diseases** such as **obesity, diabetes**, and **hypertension**. In addition, financial insecurity often leads to higher levels of **chronic stress**, which further exacerbates health conditions by affecting the body's immune response and increasing the risk of cardiovascular diseases.

Income also affects healthcare access. While wealthier individuals can afford private health insurance or out-of-pocket medical expenses, low-income individuals may delay or forgo medical treatment due to cost concerns. This delay in care often results in the progression of preventable diseases, leading to worse outcomes over time. Studies have shown that **uninsured individuals** or those underinsured are less likely to receive preventive services, such as **vaccinations, cancer screenings**, and regular **check-ups**, increasing their risk for severe health issues.

Education and Health Literacy

Education is another key determinant of health. Higher levels of education are associated with better health literacy, which refers to a person's ability to understand and use health information to make informed decisions. People with higher education levels are more likely to engage in healthy behaviors, such as **exercise, smoking cessation**, and following medical advice.

Educational attainment is strongly linked to income, but it also independently affects health. For instance, more educated individuals are better able to navigate the healthcare system, understand medication instructions, and adhere to treatment plans. They are also more likely to seek preventive care, which reduces the likelihood of developing serious health conditions.

Conversely, those with lower levels of education are at greater risk for unhealthy behaviors, such as **tobacco use**, **poor diet**, and **physical inactivity**, all of which increase the risk for chronic diseases like **cardiovascular disease** and **cancer**. Furthermore, individuals with limited education may be less aware of the **early symptoms** of disease, which can delay diagnosis and treatment.

In many cases, the health impacts of low education compound over time, creating a cycle of poor health that is passed from generation to generation. Children of parents with low educational attainment are more likely to grow up in environments that lack health-promoting resources, further perpetuating health disparities.

Occupational Status and Working Conditions

Occupation influences health both directly and indirectly. People in higher-status jobs often enjoy better working conditions, including lower physical demands, greater job security, and access to employer-sponsored health insurance. On the other hand, individuals in lower-status jobs, such as manual laborers or service industry workers, frequently face hazardous working conditions, limited job security, and fewer health benefits.

Occupational hazards include exposure to **toxic chemicals**, **loud noise**, **repetitive strain**, and **psychosocial stress**, all of which increase the risk of work-related injuries and chronic conditions like **musculoskeletal disorders** or **lung diseases**. For example, construction workers are at higher risk for **asbestos exposure**, which can lead to **mesothelioma** and other respiratory illnesses. Similarly, service workers who stand for long hours may develop **varicose veins**, **back pain**, and other musculoskeletal problems.

Low-wage workers also often face **irregular work schedules**, long hours, and little control over their working conditions, all of which contribute to **chronic stress**. This prolonged stress has been linked to a range of health problems, including **hypertension**, **mental health disorders**, and weakened immune function. Moreover, the lack of control over one's job can lead to a sense of **helplessness**, which is associated with poor mental health and increased risk for **depression** and **anxiety**.

Neighborhood and Environment

Where a person lives—often a direct result of their socioeconomic status—is influential in determining their health. Low-SES individuals are more likely to live in **disadvantaged neighborhoods** that expose them to greater environmental hazards, such as **air pollution, industrial waste**, and **unsafe drinking water**. These factors contribute to a higher prevalence of respiratory conditions, cardiovascular diseases, and certain cancers.

In addition to environmental exposures, disadvantaged neighborhoods often lack **essential health resources**, such as **quality healthcare facilities, grocery stores with fresh produce**, and **safe places to exercise**. This contributes to poor diet, physical inactivity, and increased rates of obesity and related diseases.

Crime and violence are also more prevalent in low-SES neighborhoods, creating a constant source of stress and limiting residents' ability to engage in outdoor physical activity. Children growing up in such environments are more likely to experience **trauma** and **chronic stress**, which can have long-term effects on their physical and mental health.

Health Disparities and Public Health

Socioeconomic status not only affects individual health outcomes but also drives **health disparities**—differences in health status and healthcare access between different populations. These disparities are most pronounced along lines of **race, ethnicity**, and **income**. For example, **African Americans** and **Hispanics** in the United States often face higher rates of chronic diseases, such as diabetes and hypertension, compared to **white Americans**. Much of this disparity is driven by differences in SES, with minorities more likely to experience poverty, lower educational attainment, and less access to healthcare.

Addressing these disparities requires **multifaceted public health approaches** that target the underlying social determinants of health. Programs that increase **access to education**, provide **affordable healthcare**, and improve **working conditions** can help reduce the health gap between low- and high-SES populations. Additionally, **policy interventions** that focus on improving neighborhood infrastructure, such as better housing, public transportation, and access to healthy food, are critical for reducing the health impacts of low socioeconomic status.

Impact of Race, Ethnicity, and Gender on Health Outcomes

Health outcomes are profoundly influenced by **race, ethnicity**, and **gender**. These social categories intersect with other factors like socioeconomic status, geography, and access to healthcare, leading to notable disparities in the prevalence of diseases, access to care, and overall health.

Race and Ethnicity

Racial and ethnic minorities often experience **poorer health outcomes** than their white counterparts. In many countries, particularly in the United States, **African**

Americans, **Hispanics**, **Native Americans**, and other minority groups suffer higher rates of chronic diseases like **diabetes, hypertension**, and **cardiovascular disease**. These disparities stem from a complex web of factors, including social determinants of health, healthcare access, and **structural racism**.

For example, **African Americans** in the U.S. have higher rates of **hypertension** and **stroke** compared to white populations, even after adjusting for socioeconomic status. This is partially due to chronic stress, driven by experiences of **discrimination** and **systemic inequalities**. Research suggests that **chronic exposure to stressors**, such as racial discrimination, contributes to higher **allostatic load**—the cumulative wear and tear on the body from stress, leading to worse health outcomes.

Hispanic populations face similar health challenges, particularly regarding access to healthcare. Many Hispanic individuals, especially those who are immigrants or non-citizens, lack **health insurance** or have limited access to preventive services. This leads to delayed diagnosis and treatment of conditions like diabetes, which is disproportionately higher in this group. In addition, Hispanic communities face language barriers that complicate their interactions with healthcare providers, leading to lower-quality care.

Native Americans experience some of the worst health disparities in the U.S. This population has high rates of **alcoholism, diabetes**, and **mental health disorders**, including **depression** and **suicide**. The historical trauma of colonization, forced displacement, and marginalization has created significant health burdens in Native American communities, compounded by inadequate healthcare resources and underfunded health systems on tribal lands.

Gender and Health Outcomes

Gender is another critical factor in shaping health outcomes. Men and women experience different health risks due to biological differences, but **social and cultural expectations** around gender roles also contribute to these disparities.

Women generally live longer than men but face specific health challenges. For instance, women are more likely to suffer from **chronic pain conditions** like **fibromyalgia, autoimmune diseases**, and **osteoporosis**. Women are also at higher risk for **mental health disorders**, such as **depression** and **anxiety**, often linked to social stressors like caregiving responsibilities and gender-based violence.

Gender disparities in healthcare are also well documented. **Women's health concerns** are often dismissed or undertreated, a phenomenon sometimes referred to as **medical gaslighting**. For example, women experiencing heart attack symptoms may not receive timely diagnosis or appropriate treatment, as their symptoms often differ from the "classic" presentation seen in men.

On the other hand, **men** are more likely to engage in **risky behaviors**, such as smoking, excessive alcohol consumption, and dangerous physical activities, which contribute to shorter lifespans. Men also tend to delay seeking medical care and are less likely to engage in preventive health behaviors, such as regular health checkups. These patterns lead to higher rates of **cardiovascular disease, accidents**, and **lung cancer** in men.

Intersectionality in Health Disparities

The concept of **intersectionality**—how different aspects of identity intersect to influence experiences—helps explain how race, ethnicity, and gender combine to produce unique health outcomes for certain groups. For example, **African American women** face compounded health risks due to both **racism** and **sexism**. They have higher rates of **maternal mortality** than any other racial or ethnic group in the U.S. This is driven by a combination of factors, including inadequate healthcare access, implicit biases among healthcare providers, and the effects of chronic stress from both racial and gender discrimination.

Latina women may face barriers to reproductive healthcare, including access to contraception and prenatal care, due to cultural stigmas, immigration status, or lack of insurance. Similarly, **transgender individuals** face significant health disparities due to both **gender identity** and **social marginalization**. They are more likely to experience **mental health issues**, **violence**, and **discrimination** in healthcare settings, which can lead to delayed or denied care.

The Role of Education and Employment in Health

Education and **employment** are two key social determinants of health, shaping access to resources, health literacy, and the ability to engage in health-promoting behaviors. Higher levels of education and stable, well-paying employment are consistently linked to better health outcomes, while lower education levels and precarious employment contribute to poorer health and increased risks of chronic diseases.

Education and Health

Education is important in determining health outcomes because it directly affects **health literacy**—the ability to obtain, process, and understand basic health information needed to make appropriate health decisions. Individuals with higher levels of education are more likely to engage in **preventive health behaviors**, such as regular physical activity, balanced diets, and not smoking. They are also more likely to understand the importance of medical screenings, vaccinations, and early detection of diseases.

For example, people with **higher education levels** are more likely to recognize the risks associated with **tobacco use** or **poor diets** and take steps to mitigate these risks. Education also fosters better communication skills, which help individuals navigate the healthcare system, ask informed questions, and advocate for their health needs.

Conversely, individuals with **lower education levels** are more likely to engage in **risky health behaviors**. They may be less aware of the long-term health consequences of smoking, poor diet, or lack of exercise. This lack of knowledge can lead to a higher prevalence of chronic diseases, such as **diabetes**, **heart disease**, and **cancer**, in less educated populations.

Education also indirectly affects health through its influence on employment opportunities. Those with higher education levels typically have better job prospects, which lead to higher incomes, greater job security, and access to **health insurance**. These factors create a **buffer** against many health risks.

Employment and Health

Employment is another critical determinant of health, influencing both **physical and mental well-being**. Individuals with stable, well-paying jobs tend to have better health outcomes than those in low-wage or unstable employment. Secure employment provides access to health insurance, paid leave, and the financial means to afford healthcare services, nutritious food, and safe living environments.

In contrast, **unemployment** or **precarious employment** is linked to **poorer health outcomes**. Unemployed individuals are more likely to experience **chronic stress**, **depression**, and **anxiety** due to financial insecurity. This stress can lead to a range of health problems, including cardiovascular diseases and weakened immune systems. Unemployment also limits access to healthcare, especially in countries where health insurance is tied to employment.

Even those with jobs may face health risks depending on the nature of their employment. **Low-wage workers** often face hazardous working conditions, long hours, and little control over their schedules, all of which contribute to poorer physical and mental health. For example, workers in manual labor or service industries are more prone to **workplace injuries**, **musculoskeletal disorders**, and **chronic stress** due to physically demanding work and job insecurity.

Furthermore, low-income workers are less likely to have access to **benefits** like paid sick leave, which forces many to work while ill, exacerbating health problems and spreading illnesses. They may also have limited access to healthcare if their jobs do not provide adequate insurance or if high deductibles prevent them from seeking timely medical care.

The Connection Between Education, Employment, and Long-Term Health

The relationship between **education** and **employment** creates a **feedback loop** that influences long-term health. Higher education levels lead to better employment opportunities, which provide the resources and stability needed to maintain good health. Conversely, individuals with less education often have fewer job opportunities, lower incomes, and less access to healthcare, perpetuating health disparities. Addressing these disparities requires policies that improve access to quality education and stable employment opportunities, which can ultimately lead to better health outcomes across populations.

CHAPTER 14: GENETIC EPIDEMIOLOGY

Heritability and Genetic Risk Factors for Disease

In **genetic epidemiology**, researchers investigate how genetic factors contribute to the development and distribution of diseases within populations. The concept of **heritability** and **genetic risk factors** is central to understanding the role genes play in disease occurrence and transmission across generations.

Heritability: The Genetic Contribution to Disease

Heritability refers to the proportion of variation in a disease or trait within a population that can be attributed to genetic differences between individuals. It is a statistical concept that helps determine how much of a particular trait—such as height, blood pressure, or disease susceptibility—can be explained by genetic variation rather than environmental factors.

Heritability is expressed as a percentage or a number between 0 and 1. A heritability score of **1** (or 100%) means that genetics entirely explain the variability of the trait in the population. A heritability score of **0** means that none of the variation is due to genetics, and environmental factors fully account for the differences.

It's important to understand that heritability does not apply to individuals, only to populations. For example, if a trait has a heritability of 0.7 (or 70%), this does not mean that 70% of a person's traits are determined by genetics. Instead, it means that 70% of the differences in that trait among people in the population are due to genetic factors, while the remaining 30% are due to environmental influences.

Diseases like **type 1 diabetes** or **cystic fibrosis** have high heritability, meaning genetics strongly influence whether someone will develop the condition. Other diseases, such as **type 2 diabetes** or **cardiovascular disease**, have more complex heritability due to the interaction between genetic predispositions and environmental or lifestyle factors.

Methods to Estimate Heritability

Researchers estimate heritability through various study designs. One common approach is to compare **monozygotic (identical) twins** and **dizygotic (fraternal) twins**. Identical twins share nearly 100% of their genetic material, while fraternal twins share about 50%, similar to regular siblings. By comparing the disease concordance (i.e., how often both twins get the disease) between these two groups, researchers can infer the relative contribution of genetics versus environment.

For example, if both identical twins in a pair develop **schizophrenia**, but only one fraternal twin in a pair does, researchers conclude that schizophrenia has a strong genetic component. However, if both types of twins show similar rates of disease concordance, environmental factors are likely to have a larger role.

Another method is **family studies**, where researchers look at how diseases cluster in families. If a disease is more common among close relatives than in the general population, this suggests a genetic component. However, family studies must account for shared environments, as families often live in similar conditions, making it harder to separate genetic from environmental influences.

Genetic Risk Factors

A **genetic risk factor** is a specific gene variant or mutation that increases an individual's likelihood of developing a disease. These risk factors can vary widely in terms of their impact. Some genetic mutations have a large effect, directly causing a disease, while others may only slightly increase the risk.

Monogenic diseases are caused by mutations in a single gene. These diseases often follow predictable inheritance patterns, such as **autosomal dominant** or **autosomal recessive** inheritance. For example, **Huntington's disease** is an autosomal dominant disorder, meaning that inheriting one copy of the mutated gene from either parent is sufficient to cause the disease. In contrast, **cystic fibrosis** is an autosomal recessive disorder, meaning an individual must inherit two copies of the mutated gene, one from each parent, to develop the disease.

Polygenic diseases, by contrast, involve multiple genes and are far more complex. **Type 2 diabetes**, **heart disease**, and **many cancers** fall into this category. In polygenic diseases, each gene contributes a small amount to the overall risk, and environmental factors often have a large role in triggering the disease. For example, while an individual may carry genetic risk factors for type 2 diabetes, lifestyle choices like diet and exercise significantly influence whether they will actually develop the condition.

Genome-Wide Association Studies (GWAS)

One way scientists identify genetic risk factors for complex diseases is through **genome-wide association studies (GWAS)**. GWAS involves scanning the genomes of large groups of people to look for **single nucleotide polymorphisms (SNPs)**—tiny genetic variations that occur at a single position in the genome. These SNPs are then compared between individuals with a disease and those without it.

For example, a GWAS might identify that people with certain SNPs on chromosome 9 have a higher likelihood of developing heart disease than those without these SNPs. While these genetic variations don't directly cause the disease, they indicate regions of the genome that may harbor important genes involved in disease pathways. GWAS has been successful in uncovering many genetic risk factors for diseases like **type 2 diabetes**, **Alzheimer's disease**, and **breast cancer**.

Gene-Environment Interaction

While genetics can significantly influence disease risk, it is essential to consider the interaction between genes and the environment. Many diseases, particularly common chronic conditions, result from **gene-environment interactions**, where environmental exposures (such as diet, pollution, or physical activity) modify the effect of genetic predispositions.

For example, someone may carry genetic risk factors for **obesity**, but they may not become obese if they maintain a healthy diet and regular exercise routine. Similarly, individuals with a genetic predisposition to **lung cancer** may increase their risk dramatically if they are exposed to **cigarette smoke**.

This interaction highlights the complexity of predicting disease risk based solely on genetic information. Even with high genetic risk, lifestyle and environmental interventions can still have a significant impact on preventing disease.

Applications in Personalized Medicine

Understanding genetic risk factors has paved the way for **personalized medicine**, where healthcare is tailored to an individual's genetic makeup. For instance, genetic testing can identify individuals with **BRCA1** or **BRCA2** mutations, which significantly increase the risk of **breast and ovarian cancers**. Armed with this knowledge, patients can make informed decisions about preventive measures, such as enhanced screening or even **prophylactic surgery** to reduce cancer risk.

Similarly, pharmacogenomics—how genes affect a person's response to drugs— allows for personalized treatment plans. Genetic testing can help predict which medications will be most effective or carry the fewest side effects for specific individuals, leading to more effective disease management.

Gene-Environment Interactions

Gene-environment interactions occur when environmental factors influence the expression of genetic traits, or when genetic predispositions affect how individuals respond to environmental exposures. This concept is critical in understanding how complex diseases develop because most common diseases result from a combination of both **genetic** and **environmental** factors. While some individuals may carry genetic risk factors, their likelihood of developing a disease can vary significantly depending on lifestyle choices, exposures, and living conditions.

How Gene-Environment Interactions Work

A **gene-environment interaction** refers to a situation where the effect of an environmental exposure on disease risk differs depending on an individual's genotype. Conversely, it can also refer to a genetic predisposition that is only triggered or amplified by certain environmental exposures. This interaction complicates the process of predicting disease risk based solely on genetic or environmental factors alone, as both need to be considered in concert to understand health outcomes fully.

Take **lung cancer** as an example. Smoking is a major environmental risk factor for lung cancer, but not everyone who smokes develops the disease. Some individuals have genetic variations that make them more susceptible to the carcinogenic effects of tobacco. For these individuals, their genetic makeup amplifies the harmful effects of smoking, increasing their risk. On the other hand, someone with the same genetic predisposition who never smokes may have a much lower risk of developing lung cancer.

Another example is **skin cancer**. Individuals with fair skin, often due to specific genetic traits, are at higher risk for developing skin cancer, especially if they experience excessive exposure to ultraviolet (UV) radiation from the sun. Their genetic predisposition makes them more vulnerable to the effects of sun exposure, while people with darker skin may have a natural protective factor against UV damage, even in similar environmental conditions.

Complex Diseases and Gene-Environment Interactions

Many **complex diseases**, such as **cardiovascular disease**, **type 2 diabetes**, and **obesity**, arise from the interplay between genes and environmental factors. **Obesity**, for instance, has a genetic component, with certain gene variants, such as **FTO**, associated with a higher likelihood of becoming obese. However, individuals carrying these genetic risk factors may not become obese if they live in an environment that promotes healthy eating and physical activity. This demonstrates how environmental modifications can mitigate genetic risks.

Similarly, **type 2 diabetes** results from both genetic susceptibility and environmental factors like diet, exercise, and body weight. While a person may have genes that predispose them to insulin resistance, maintaining a healthy lifestyle can prevent the expression of these genes or delay the onset of the disease. Conversely, an unhealthy diet high in sugar and fats can trigger the disease in someone with a genetic predisposition.

Cardiovascular disease is another condition influenced by gene-environment interactions. Genetic factors may predispose individuals to high cholesterol or hypertension, but factors like smoking, diet, and exercise are important in whether or not these conditions lead to heart disease.

The Importance of Studying Gene-Environment Interactions

Understanding gene-environment interactions is essential for several reasons. First, it helps **identify high-risk groups** within populations. By recognizing which individuals carry certain genetic risk factors and identifying the environmental exposures that exacerbate those risks, public health interventions can be more precisely targeted.

For example, people with a family history of **breast cancer** due to mutations in the **BRCA1** or **BRCA2** genes may benefit from more frequent screenings or preventive interventions, especially if they are exposed to environmental factors like high-dose radiation, which could further increase their cancer risk.

Second, studying these interactions can guide **preventive strategies**. In many cases, knowing the environmental triggers that affect genetic predispositions can lead to targeted public health policies. **Smoking cessation programs, nutritional guidelines**, and **physical activity recommendations** can be tailored to individuals based on their genetic profiles to prevent disease.

Third, gene-environment interaction studies provide insights into the **biological mechanisms** that underlie disease development. For instance, understanding how certain genes are activated or suppressed by environmental factors can lead to **new drug targets** or **therapeutic interventions** that modify disease progression. This is the foundation of **precision medicine**, which aims to create personalized treatment and prevention strategies based on an individual's genetic makeup and environmental exposures.

Challenges in Gene-Environment Interaction Research

Research into gene-environment interactions faces several challenges. One of the main difficulties is the **complexity of interactions** between multiple genes and a wide range of environmental factors. Diseases like type 2 diabetes involve dozens, if not hundreds, of genes, each interacting with lifestyle factors like diet and physical activity in different ways. Isolating the specific contribution of each factor is a difficult task.

Additionally, **data collection** can be challenging. Gene-environment interaction studies require large sample sizes to capture the variability in genetic and environmental exposures across populations. Accurate measurement of environmental exposures, such as diet, exercise, pollutants, or stress, is also essential but can be difficult to achieve over long periods.

Moving Forward: Personalized Medicine

The study of gene-environment interactions is a critical piece of the puzzle in the movement toward **personalized medicine**. By understanding how genes and environments work together to influence disease, healthcare providers can offer more tailored advice. For example, someone with a genetic predisposition to **high**

cholesterol might benefit from more aggressive lifestyle interventions, such as a low-fat diet and regular physical activity, even before their cholesterol levels rise.

Pharmacogenomics, the study of how genes influence a person's response to drugs, is another growing field in personalized medicine. This approach considers genetic variability when prescribing medications, allowing for more effective treatment with fewer side effects.

Population Genetics in Epidemiologic Studies

Population genetics explores the distribution of genetic variation within populations and how these genetic differences affect traits, including susceptibility to diseases. In **epidemiologic studies**, population genetics is essential for understanding how genes influence health and disease on a broader scale. This field helps researchers identify genetic risk factors, track the spread of genetic traits through populations, and understand the evolutionary forces shaping human health.

Genetic Variation in Populations

At the core of population genetics is **genetic variation**, which refers to the differences in DNA sequences between individuals. This variation can manifest in small changes like **single nucleotide polymorphisms (SNPs)** or larger structural changes in the genome. SNPs are the most common type of genetic variation, where a single nucleotide in the DNA sequence differs between individuals.

These genetic differences can influence how individuals respond to environmental exposures, medications, or their susceptibility to diseases. For example, a population with a high frequency of a gene variant that protects against **malaria**, such as the **sickle cell trait**, may have a lower incidence of the disease but also a higher prevalence of **sickle cell disease** under certain genetic combinations.

Population stratification—the presence of genetic subgroups within a population —can complicate epidemiologic studies. Differences in allele frequencies between subgroups can lead to misleading associations between genes and diseases unless properly accounted for. For this reason, epidemiologists must consider **ancestry** and **genetic background** when studying genetic contributions to diseases.

Hardy-Weinberg Equilibrium and Population Genetics

One of the key concepts in population genetics is the **Hardy-Weinberg equilibrium** (HWE), which provides a mathematical framework to describe the distribution of alleles in a population. According to HWE, allele and genotype frequencies will remain constant from generation to generation in the absence of **evolutionary forces** like **mutation**, **selection**, **genetic drift**, or **migration**.

In epidemiologic studies, HWE is often used as a baseline to determine if a population is evolving or if certain alleles are under selection due to disease pressures. For example, deviations from HWE in a population might indicate **selective pressures** acting on a gene related to disease resistance or susceptibility.

Genetic Drift, Migration, and Disease Patterns

Genetic drift is the random fluctuation of allele frequencies from one generation to the next, particularly in small populations. This can lead to the loss or fixation of alleles over time, affecting disease susceptibility within populations. In larger populations, drift has less of an impact, but in isolated or small groups, it can result in the persistence of rare diseases. For example, **Tay-Sachs disease** is more common in certain populations due to genetic drift and **founder effects**.

Migration also is important in shaping the genetic landscape of populations. When individuals migrate and interbreed with new populations, they introduce new genetic variants. This gene flow can affect the distribution of disease-associated alleles. For instance, as populations with European ancestry migrated to the Americas, they brought genes associated with diseases like **cystic fibrosis** or **hemochromatosis**, changing the genetic disease profile in these regions.

Evolutionary Pressures and Disease Susceptibility

Population genetics helps explain why certain genetic traits or disease susceptibilities are more common in some populations than others. **Natural selection** has favored some genetic traits that increase survival under specific environmental conditions. For instance, the **lactase persistence** allele, which allows adults to digest lactose, is more common in populations with a long history of dairy consumption.

Similarly, the high prevalence of **sickle cell trait** in parts of Africa is a result of evolutionary pressure. The trait provides resistance to malaria, giving individuals with one copy of the gene a survival advantage in malaria-endemic regions. However, having two copies of the gene leads to **sickle cell disease**, illustrating the complex balance of genetic traits in populations.

Applications in Epidemiologic Studies

Population genetics is essential in genome-wide association studies where researchers examine the genomes of large groups of people to identify genetic variants associated with diseases. GWAS helps uncover **single nucleotide polymorphisms (SNPs)** or other genetic markers that may contribute to disease risk. By comparing genetic variations between those with and without a specific disease, scientists can pinpoint the regions of the genome that may influence susceptibility.

However, one of the challenges in GWAS is **population stratification**, where differences in genetic ancestry between subgroups within a study population can create spurious associations between genetic markers and disease. For example, if one subgroup has both a higher frequency of a particular SNP and a higher rate of the disease being studied, researchers may falsely attribute the disease risk to that SNP, when in reality, the association is due to ancestry rather than a true genetic effect. Adjusting for population structure through methods like **principal component analysis (PCA)** is critical to avoid these false positives.

Genetic Epidemiology and Global Disease Patterns

Population genetics also is important in understanding how genetic susceptibility to diseases varies across different geographic and ethnic groups. Certain diseases are more prevalent in some populations due to historical selection pressures, migration patterns, or genetic drift. For instance, the **APOE ε4 allele**, a genetic risk factor for **Alzheimer's disease**, has different frequencies across populations, contributing to variations in Alzheimer's disease prevalence globally.

In diseases like **type 2 diabetes**, researchers have found that certain populations, such as **South Asians** and **Native Americans**, have higher genetic susceptibility, likely due to evolutionary adaptations to their ancestral environments. These populations historically thrived in environments where food was scarce, but as they have transitioned to more modern, high-calorie diets, the genetic predispositions that once helped conserve energy have increased their risk for metabolic disorders.

Precision Medicine and Population Genetics

Population genetics is also foundational to the development of **precision medicine**, which aims to tailor healthcare based on an individual's genetic background. As scientists identify genetic variants that influence how individuals respond to specific treatments or environmental exposures, medical interventions can become more personalized.

For example, individuals with certain genetic variants metabolize drugs differently, making them more or less responsive to specific medications. **Pharmacogenomics**, a field within precision medicine, uses genetic information to predict drug response and guide treatment decisions, helping to minimize adverse drug reactions and optimize therapy. A well-known example is the testing for variants in the **CYP450** genes, which affect the metabolism of drugs like **warfarin** and **antidepressants**. By considering genetic differences, clinicians can prescribe more effective and safer dosages.

The Role of Large-Scale Biobanks

Large-scale **biobanks**—repositories that store genetic, health, and lifestyle information from large numbers of people—have become invaluable resources for genetic epidemiology. By combining genetic data with health records, researchers can study the relationships between genes, environment, and disease outcomes across diverse populations. Biobanks like the **UK Biobank** or the **All of Us Research Program** in the U.S. are enabling researchers to study a wide range of diseases, from cancer to cardiovascular conditions, with unprecedented precision.

These resources are particularly useful for understanding gene-environment interactions, as they provide detailed information about both genetic makeup and environmental exposures. For example, researchers can study how a genetic predisposition to **hypertension** interacts with lifestyle factors like **diet**, **exercise**, and **salt intake** to influence the development of high blood pressure.

Ethical Considerations in Population Genetics

As genetic data becomes more integrated into epidemiologic research, **ethical issues** arise. One major concern is **genetic privacy** and the potential misuse of genetic information. For example, individuals might be concerned about **genetic discrimination** in employment or insurance if their genetic data reveals a higher risk for certain diseases. To address these concerns, policies like the **Genetic Information Nondiscrimination Act (GINA)** in the U.S. have been implemented to protect individuals from such discrimination based on their genetic information.

Another ethical consideration is **equity in genetic research**. Historically, genetic studies have disproportionately focused on populations of **European ancestry**, which means that the benefits of genetic discoveries—such as new treatments or risk predictions—are often less applicable to non-European populations. Increasing diversity in genetic research is essential to ensure that the advances in precision medicine benefit all populations equitably.

CHAPTER 15: EPIDEMIOLOGY AND GLOBAL HEALTH

Emerging and Re-Emerging Infectious Diseases

Emerging and re-emerging infectious diseases present a major challenge to global health, impacting populations in both high-income and low-income countries. These diseases are caused by **pathogens**—bacteria, viruses, fungi, or parasites—that can spread between individuals, often across international borders, due to increased travel, trade, and environmental changes. **Emerging infectious diseases (EIDs)** refer to diseases that are newly recognized in a population, while **re-emerging infectious diseases** are those that were once under control but have resurfaced due to various factors like pathogen evolution, changes in population immunity, or breakdowns in public health infrastructure.

Emerging Infectious Diseases

Emerging infectious diseases can arise from **newly discovered pathogens**, **zoonotic spillover events**, or previously unrecognized forms of existing pathogens. These diseases often spread rapidly and can have widespread consequences.

One recent example of an emerging disease is **COVID-19**, caused by the novel **SARS-CoV-2** virus. First identified in Wuhan, China, in late 2019, the virus quickly spread worldwide, leading to a global pandemic. The emergence of SARS-CoV-2 was linked to zoonotic transmission, where the virus likely jumped from animals to humans, highlighting the close relationship between human health and wildlife. In addition to its direct health impact, COVID-19 disrupted economies, overwhelmed healthcare systems, and highlighted gaps in pandemic preparedness.

Another notable example is **Ebola virus disease**, which has caused multiple outbreaks in West Africa and other regions since its discovery in 1976. The 2014-2016 Ebola outbreak in West Africa was particularly devastating, resulting in over 11,000 deaths. Ebola is a **zoonotic virus**, meaning it is transmitted from animals to humans, often through contact with infected wildlife. The disease spreads through direct contact with bodily fluids and can lead to severe hemorrhagic fever with high fatality rates. In the case of Ebola, delayed recognition of the outbreak, insufficient healthcare infrastructure, and lack of rapid containment measures contributed to its rapid spread.

Another emerging disease of concern is **Zika virus**, which made headlines in 2015 when it spread across the Americas, causing widespread outbreaks. Zika is transmitted primarily by **Aedes mosquitoes**, and while the virus typically causes mild symptoms, it can have devastating effects on pregnancy, leading to **microcephaly** and other birth defects in infants. The Zika outbreak raised global awareness of the importance of mosquito control and the need for better surveillance systems in areas where vector-borne diseases are common.

Factors Driving the Emergence of Infectious Diseases

Several factors contribute to the emergence of new infectious diseases. **Urbanization** and the growth of megacities place people in closer proximity, increasing the chances of disease transmission. As people encroach on **natural habitats**, they come into contact with wildlife, increasing the likelihood of zoonotic spillovers. **Deforestation** and agricultural expansion also displace animals, pushing them closer to human settlements and allowing pathogens to jump species.

Globalization is critical in the spread of emerging diseases. Increased air travel and international trade allow pathogens to move across borders more easily. A disease that originates in one part of the world can now reach distant continents in a matter of days. **Climate change** is another factor that influences the spread of infectious diseases. Warmer temperatures can expand the habitats of disease-carrying vectors, such as mosquitoes, leading to the spread of diseases like **dengue**, **malaria**, and **Zika** into new regions that were previously unaffected.

Re-Emerging Infectious Diseases

Re-emerging diseases are those that were previously controlled or nearly eradicated but have resurfaced due to changing conditions, **pathogen evolution**, or lapses in public health measures. These diseases often highlight the fragility of public health systems and the ongoing need for vigilance, even after significant progress in disease control.

One well-known example of a re-emerging disease is **tuberculosis (TB)**. TB is an ancient disease that once seemed to be on the decline, but the emergence of **multidrug-resistant tuberculosis (MDR-TB)** and **extensively drug-resistant tuberculosis (XDR-TB)** has complicated efforts to control it. Drug-resistant TB arises from incomplete or improper use of antibiotics, which allows the bacteria to evolve and become resistant to treatment. In many low-resource settings, limited access to healthcare and medications exacerbates the spread of TB, particularly in areas with high rates of **HIV/AIDS**, as co-infection with HIV weakens the immune system and increases the risk of developing active TB.

Measles is another re-emerging disease that has seen a resurgence in recent years, particularly in high-income countries where it was once considered nearly eradicated. The rise of **vaccine hesitancy** and the spread of misinformation about vaccines have led to declines in **measles vaccination coverage**, allowing the disease to spread among unvaccinated populations. Measles is highly contagious, and outbreaks can spread rapidly in communities with low vaccination rates, leading to severe complications like pneumonia and encephalitis, particularly in young children.

Malaria, once brought under control in many parts of the world, has also experienced a resurgence in some areas. **Insecticide resistance** in mosquitoes and **drug resistance** in the parasite that causes malaria have made it more difficult to control the disease. Additionally, changing environmental conditions, such as increased rainfall and warmer temperatures, are expanding the range of mosquitoes that carry malaria, contributing to its re-emergence in regions where it had previously been eliminated.

Addressing Emerging and Re-Emerging Diseases

The emergence and re-emergence of infectious diseases underscore the need for **robust global health systems** capable of rapid detection, containment, and response. Surveillance systems, such as the **Global Outbreak Alert and Response Network**, are influential in monitoring disease outbreaks and coordinating international efforts to contain them. In addition, investments in **vaccine development**, **public health infrastructure**, and **vector control programs** are essential to prevent the spread of infectious diseases.

Strengthening **healthcare systems** in low- and middle-income countries is also critical, as these regions are often disproportionately affected by emerging and re-emerging diseases. Global cooperation, research, and funding are needed to build capacity in these areas, enabling quicker responses to outbreaks and improving disease control efforts. Public health campaigns that focus on **improving vaccination rates**, **promoting hygiene**, and **strengthening infection control measures** can also help prevent the spread of diseases that are prone to re-emerging.

Global Surveillance Systems (WHO, CDC, etc.)

Global surveillance systems are vital in detecting, tracking, and responding to infectious diseases across the world. These systems, led by organizations like the **World Health Organization (WHO)** and the **Centers for Disease Control and Prevention (CDC)**, work to monitor disease trends, identify emerging threats, and coordinate international responses to outbreaks. Effective surveillance is crucial for preventing the spread of infectious diseases, especially in an interconnected world where pathogens can cross borders quickly.

The World Health Organization (WHO)

The **World Health Organization (WHO)** coordinates international public health efforts and provides guidance on disease control measures. One of the WHO's key tools for disease surveillance is the **Global Outbreak Alert and Response Network (GOARN)**, which is a network of technical institutions, public health agencies, and laboratories that work together to identify and respond to outbreaks.

GOARN enables rapid information sharing and collaboration across countries. When a disease outbreak is detected, GOARN mobilizes experts, resources, and technical support to the affected area to help contain and manage the outbreak. This was critical during the **Ebola outbreak** in West Africa, where GOARN had a key role in coordinating the international response.

The WHO also maintains the **International Health Regulations (IHR)**, a legal framework that requires countries to report certain disease outbreaks and public health events. The IHR helps ensure that countries are transparent about emerging health threats and are prepared to collaborate with the international community in controlling diseases.

The Centers for Disease Control and Prevention (CDC)

The **Centers for Disease Control and Prevention (CDC)** is a leading national public health institute in the United States but also is significant in global health surveillance. The CDC operates **Global Disease Detection (GDD)** centers around the world, which monitor and respond to infectious diseases in different regions. These centers provide critical early warning systems for disease outbreaks and offer expertise in laboratory diagnostics, epidemiology, and health system strengthening.

The CDC's **Epidemic Intelligence Service (EIS)** trains disease detectives who investigate outbreaks worldwide, including diseases like **cholera**, **influenza**, and **Zika virus**. EIS officers are deployed to assist in disease investigations, collect data, and help implement containment measures during public health emergencies.

The Global Influenza Surveillance and Response System (GISRS)

One of the most important disease surveillance networks is the **Global Influenza Surveillance and Response System (GISRS)**, coordinated by the WHO. GISRS monitors the spread of **influenza viruses** and provides critical data on emerging flu strains. This information is used to inform the composition of seasonal **influenza vaccines** and prepare for potential flu pandemics.

GISRS includes a network of over 150 national laboratories worldwide that collect and analyze flu virus samples. The system tracks flu virus mutations, which helps experts determine which strains are most likely to circulate in the upcoming flu season. This surveillance network has been instrumental in responding to flu pandemics, such as the **H1N1 pandemic** in 2009.

Challenges in Global Surveillance

Despite the effectiveness of global surveillance systems, there are significant challenges. In many low- and middle-income countries, **lack of infrastructure** and **limited healthcare resources** hinder surveillance efforts. Poor access to diagnostic tools and laboratory facilities can delay the detection of outbreaks, allowing diseases to spread before they are identified.

Additionally, **political instability** and **conflict** in some regions make it difficult to collect accurate data or implement public health interventions. Outbreaks in war zones, refugee camps, or regions with weak governance often go unreported or are poorly managed, increasing the risk of global spread.

Data sharing between countries and organizations can also be a challenge. Some governments may be reluctant to report disease outbreaks due to fears of economic consequences, such as travel restrictions or trade bans. This can lead to delayed responses and make it harder to contain outbreaks before they become widespread.

Strengthening Global Surveillance

To strengthen global disease surveillance, there is a need for more **investment in health infrastructure** and **capacity building** in low-resource settings. Training healthcare workers, improving laboratory networks, and enhancing real-time data collection are critical steps to ensure rapid detection and response to emerging health threats.

Additionally, fostering better **international collaboration** and transparency is crucial. Public health should take precedence over political or economic concerns, and countries must prioritize the timely sharing of data on emerging diseases. The COVID-19 pandemic underscored the importance of global surveillance systems and the need for coordinated international responses to public health emergencies.

Epidemiology of Pandemics: Historical and Modern Examples

The **epidemiology of pandemics** provides insight into how infectious diseases spread across populations, both historically and in modern times. Pandemics, defined as outbreaks of infectious diseases that occur on a global scale, have shaped human history, influencing mortality, migration, economies, and societies. Understanding the epidemiologic patterns of pandemics—how diseases emerge, spread, peak, and decline—enables public health officials to develop strategies to mitigate their impact. Both historical and modern examples, from the **Black Death** to **COVID-19**, offer valuable lessons for managing future outbreaks.

The Black Death (1347–1351)

The **Black Death**, one of the deadliest pandemics in human history, swept through Europe, Asia, and North Africa in the 14th century. Caused by the bacterium **Yersinia pestis**, which is transmitted through flea bites, the Black Death is believed to have originated in Central Asia before spreading westward via trade routes.

The disease reached Europe in 1347, devastating populations with high mortality rates—killing an estimated 25–30 million people in Europe alone, approximately 30–60% of the continent's population. The epidemic spread rapidly, aided by high population densities in cities and poor sanitation. The **bubonic form** of the plague, characterized by swollen lymph nodes (buboes), was the most common, but **pneumonic plague**, which spreads through respiratory droplets, also had a role in its rapid transmission.

From an epidemiological perspective, the **lack of immunity** in populations, combined with **unsanitary living conditions**, allowed the plague to spread uncontrollably. The Black Death changed the demographic landscape of Europe, leading to significant labor shortages, shifts in social structures, and even contributing to the decline of feudalism.

The Spanish Flu (1918–1919)

The **Spanish Flu**, caused by an **H1N1 influenza virus**, was another catastrophic pandemic, infecting about a third of the world's population and killing an estimated 50–100 million people. Unlike previous influenza outbreaks, the Spanish Flu disproportionately affected young, healthy adults between the ages of 20 and 40, with an unusually high **case fatality rate** in this age group.

The first wave of the Spanish Flu, which began in the spring of 1918, was relatively mild. However, the second wave in the fall of 1918 was far more severe, characterized by **cytokine storms**—an overreaction of the immune system—that caused severe respiratory distress and death in many patients. This second wave was particularly deadly because the virus had mutated, becoming more virulent.

The Spanish Flu spread through **crowded conditions**, including **military camps** during World War I, and further accelerated by the movement of troops. The pandemic is notable for the speed of its spread and the global reach, facilitated by increased travel and the movement of people due to the war. Public health responses were hampered by limited knowledge of the virus, lack of vaccines, and ineffective treatment options.

Epidemiologically, the Spanish Flu highlighted the importance of **public health measures** like **quarantine**, **social distancing**, and **isolation** in controlling the spread of highly infectious diseases. Despite these measures, the global death toll was immense, and the pandemic significantly strained healthcare systems and economies.

HIV/AIDS Pandemic (1981–Present)

The **HIV/AIDS pandemic**, caused by the **human immunodeficiency virus (HIV)**, has been ongoing since it was first recognized in the early 1980s. Unlike other pandemics that spread rapidly and then subside, HIV/AIDS has been a slow-burning pandemic that has affected millions of people over the past four decades.

According to the **World Health Organization (WHO)**, over 36 million people have died from AIDS-related illnesses, and around 38 million people are currently living with HIV.

HIV is primarily transmitted through **sexual contact, blood transfusions,** and **needle sharing,** as well as from **mother to child** during childbirth or breastfeeding. The virus attacks the immune system, specifically **CD4 cells,** leaving the body vulnerable to opportunistic infections and cancers. Without treatment, HIV progresses to **AIDS,** which is fatal.

The spread of HIV/AIDS has been shaped by **social and behavioral factors,** such as sexual practices, stigma, and drug use, as well as structural factors like **access to healthcare** and **socioeconomic conditions.** The pandemic has disproportionately affected marginalized populations, including **men who have sex with men (MSM), sex workers, intravenous drug users,** and **people in low-income countries,** particularly in **Sub-Saharan Africa.**

The introduction of **antiretroviral therapy (ART)** in the mid-1990s significantly changed the epidemiology of HIV/AIDS by transforming it from a death sentence to a manageable chronic condition. However, the pandemic continues to pose challenges due to **inequalities in healthcare access, stigma,** and the need for **lifelong treatment.**

SARS (2002–2003)

The **Severe Acute Respiratory Syndrome (SARS)** outbreak of 2002-2003 was caused by a **coronavirus (SARS-CoV-1)** and was one of the first significant global outbreaks of the 21st century. It originated in **Guangdong, China,** and rapidly spread to over 30 countries, with more than 8,000 reported cases and nearly 800 deaths.

SARS was primarily spread through **respiratory droplets** and had a relatively high case fatality rate of around 9.6%. The disease caused **severe pneumonia** and other respiratory complications. Unlike more contagious viruses like influenza, SARS was less easily transmitted because people were most infectious after symptoms appeared, allowing public health officials to identify and isolate cases more effectively.

The global response to SARS demonstrated the importance of **rapid containment measures.** The **WHO** and national health agencies implemented **contact tracing, isolation,** and **quarantine** procedures, which successfully halted the spread of the virus. SARS was also a turning point in global health, highlighting the need for **improved surveillance systems** and better preparedness for future pandemics.

H1N1 Pandemic (2009)

In 2009, the world experienced another **H1N1 influenza pandemic**, but this time the virus was less deadly than the Spanish Flu. The H1N1 virus, also known as **swine flu**, originated in pigs and was transmitted to humans. It spread rapidly, infecting millions of people worldwide, but the **case fatality rate** was relatively low compared to previous pandemics.

The H1N1 pandemic primarily affected **young people**, including children and young adults, with relatively mild symptoms for most individuals. However, some groups, such as **pregnant women, people with underlying health conditions**, and **the elderly**, experienced more severe illness.

The **CDC** and **WHO** responded quickly by coordinating vaccination campaigns and public health measures, reducing the pandemic's overall impact. H1N1 marked a shift in pandemic preparedness, as many countries had established **pandemic response plans** and **stockpiled vaccines** following the SARS outbreak.

COVID-19 Pandemic (2019–Present)

The **COVID-19 pandemic** is the most recent and one of the most disruptive global health crises of the modern era. Caused by the novel **SARS-CoV-2** virus, COVID-19 first emerged in **Wuhan, China**, in late 2019 and spread rapidly worldwide. By early 2020, the WHO declared it a global pandemic.

COVID-19 is primarily transmitted through **respiratory droplets** and **airborne transmission**, making it highly contagious. The disease manifests in a range of symptoms, from mild respiratory illness to severe **pneumonia, acute respiratory distress syndrome (ARDS)**, and **multi-organ failure**. The pandemic has caused over **6 million deaths** globally and led to unprecedented social, economic, and healthcare challenges.

The pandemic's **epidemiology** is marked by multiple waves of infection, driven by the emergence of new **variants** like **Delta** and **Omicron**, which have different levels of transmissibility and immune evasion. The rapid development and distribution of **COVID-19 vaccines**—such as the **Pfizer-BioNTech** and **Moderna mRNA vaccines**—have been critical in reducing severe illness and death, although vaccine distribution has been uneven, particularly in low-income countries.

COVID-19 has highlighted the importance of **global cooperation, public health infrastructure**, and **surveillance systems** in pandemic preparedness. Public health measures like **social distancing, mask-wearing**, and **quarantine** were widely implemented but also became points of political and social contention. The pandemic has stressed healthcare systems globally and exposed inequalities in access to care, vaccines, and resources.

Lessons from Pandemic Epidemiology

Each of these pandemics—whether it be the **Black Death, Spanish Flu, HIV/ AIDS, SARS, H1N1,** or **COVID-19**—provides important lessons for the future. First, **early detection** and **rapid response** are critical to containing the spread of infectious diseases. Delays in recognizing outbreaks, whether due to lack of surveillance or inadequate infrastructure, often lead to more severe outcomes.

Second, the **global nature** of modern pandemics requires coordinated international responses. Pathogens do not respect borders, and a disease that starts in one country can quickly spread across the world. Global surveillance systems, such as the **Global Outbreak Alert and Response Network (GOARN)**, have a key role in identifying and responding to pandemics.

Third, pandemics disproportionately affect vulnerable populations, such as those in **low-income countries, marginalized communities,** or with **limited access to healthcare**. Addressing these disparities is critical for controlling the spread of diseases and ensuring that the most vulnerable are protected. Pandemics expose weaknesses in health systems, particularly in low-resource settings where healthcare infrastructure may be inadequate to handle large-scale outbreaks. Ensuring equitable access to **healthcare, vaccines,** and **medications** must be a priority in future pandemic preparedness efforts.

Globalization and Urbanization

Pandemics are also facilitated by **globalization** and **urbanization**, where the movement of people, goods, and animals across borders increases the potential for disease spread. Global travel networks allow diseases to move quickly between countries, while dense urban environments provide ideal conditions for infectious agents to spread among large populations. In modern times, diseases like **SARS, H1N1,** and **COVID-19** have demonstrated how quickly pathogens can cross borders due to global travel and trade.

Urbanization has a role in creating conditions ripe for transmission. **High population densities**, often combined with **poor sanitation** and **overcrowded living conditions**, allow diseases to spread rapidly in cities. This was evident during the **Black Death** and remains true today in many low- and middle-income countries where access to clean water, sanitation, and healthcare is limited. The rapid expansion of megacities increases the risk of outbreaks and requires public health systems to adapt to these changing environments.

Vaccination and Immunity

Vaccination has been one of the most effective tools in combating pandemics. The successful eradication of **smallpox** and the near-elimination of diseases like **polio** demonstrate how vaccines can prevent large-scale outbreaks. However, achieving high levels of vaccination coverage is essential for creating **herd immunity**, which prevents the spread of infectious diseases even to those who are not vaccinated.

The success of vaccination programs in pandemics like **H1N1** and **COVID-19** is a testament to the importance of rapid vaccine development and distribution. However, **vaccine hesitancy**, misinformation, and logistical challenges have undermined efforts in some regions. The COVID-19 pandemic revealed significant disparities in vaccine access, with high-income countries securing vaccines early while lower-income nations faced delays. This unequal distribution can prolong pandemics by allowing the virus to continue circulating and evolving into new variants.

The development of **mRNA vaccines** during the COVID-19 pandemic has opened new avenues for rapid vaccine deployment in future pandemics. This technology enables the quick adaptation of vaccines to target new strains or emerging pathogens, making it a crucial tool for future preparedness.

Public Health Infrastructure

Pandemics have shown the importance of robust **public health infrastructure**. Systems for **disease surveillance**, **contact tracing**, and **laboratory testing** are critical for early detection and response to emerging threats. Countries with well-funded public health systems were generally better able to respond to pandemics, while those with underfunded systems faced significant challenges in controlling outbreaks.

The **Epidemic Intelligence Service (EIS)** of the CDC, the **Global Influenza Surveillance and Response System (GISRS)**, and the WHO's **GOARN** are examples of systems designed to monitor and respond to pandemics on a global scale. These networks facilitate information sharing, coordinate responses, and mobilize resources during pandemics, but they need continuous investment and expansion to keep pace with evolving global threats.

Public health measures such as **quarantine, social distancing, mask-wearing,** and **travel restrictions** have been used throughout history to control the spread of infectious diseases. These measures have proven effective in slowing transmission, though they can also be politically and socially challenging. The COVID-19 pandemic, in particular, highlighted the importance of clear and consistent communication from public health officials to gain public compliance with health directives.

Preparedness and Future Outlook

Pandemics will continue to be a threat as long as humans interact closely with animals, the environment, and each other. **Zoonotic diseases**—those that spread from animals to humans—will likely remain a primary source of emerging infectious diseases, as seen with **HIV/AIDS, SARS, Ebola**, and **COVID-19**. Preventing future pandemics will require investment in **veterinary epidemiology**, **environmental monitoring**, and **One Health** approaches that recognize the interconnectedness of human, animal, and environmental health.

Pandemic preparedness requires international cooperation, political will, and financial investment. Countries must invest in **surge capacity** for healthcare systems, ensure the availability of **personal protective equipment (PPE)**, and maintain stockpiles of **essential medications**. Additionally, governments must prioritize **research and development** of vaccines and treatments for a wide range of potential pathogens, including those that currently pose limited threats but have the potential to cause global outbreaks.

Global initiatives like the **Coalition for Epidemic Preparedness Innovations (CEPI)**, which focuses on accelerating the development of vaccines for emerging infectious diseases, will be important in future pandemic preparedness. The lessons from past pandemics, particularly COVID-19, emphasize the need for resilient healthcare systems capable of responding quickly to new threats.

Vaccination Programs and Disease Eradication

Vaccination programs are one of the most effective public health tools for preventing infectious diseases and, in some cases, eradicating them. Vaccines protect individuals from contracting diseases by stimulating the immune system to recognize and fight specific pathogens. On a larger scale, widespread vaccination can significantly reduce the prevalence of a disease, and in some cases, lead to complete eradication. Disease eradication occurs when a disease is eliminated from the entire world, while **elimination** refers to the reduction of a disease to zero cases in a specific geographic area.

How Vaccination Programs Work

Vaccination programs are designed to reach large segments of the population to create **herd immunity**, where enough people are immune to a disease to prevent it from spreading. **Herd immunity** protects even those who cannot be vaccinated, such as individuals with weakened immune systems or allergies to vaccine components, by reducing their risk of being exposed to the disease.

For vaccination programs to be effective, high **coverage rates** are necessary. The proportion of the population that needs to be vaccinated to achieve herd immunity varies depending on the disease's **basic reproduction number (R0)**, which measures how contagious a disease is. For highly contagious diseases like **measles**, around 95% of the population must be vaccinated to prevent outbreaks. In contrast, for less contagious diseases like **polio**, a lower coverage rate (around 80-85%) may be sufficient to stop transmission.

Success Stories in Disease Eradication

The most successful example of a vaccination program leading to disease eradication is the eradication of **smallpox**. Through a concerted global effort led by the WHO, smallpox was declared eradicated in 1980, after a massive vaccination campaign that reached nearly every corner of the world. This was possible because **smallpox** had no animal reservoir, meaning it could not survive outside of humans, and the vaccine was highly effective in conferring long-lasting immunity.

Another ongoing eradication effort is the global campaign to eliminate **polio**. **Polio** was once a widespread and devastating disease, causing paralysis in thousands of children worldwide. Thanks to the development of effective **oral polio vaccines (OPV)** and massive global vaccination efforts, **polio** has been eliminated in most parts of the world. However, the disease remains endemic in a few countries, including **Afghanistan** and **Pakistan**, where political instability, conflict, and vaccine misinformation have slowed eradication efforts. Despite these challenges, the global effort to eradicate polio continues, with recent years showing significant progress toward reducing the number of cases.

Challenges in Vaccination Programs

While vaccines have led to the elimination and control of many diseases, there are still significant challenges to achieving global vaccination coverage. **Vaccine hesitancy** is one of the major barriers to effective vaccination programs. In recent years, misinformation and mistrust in vaccines, often spread through social media, have led to a decline in vaccination rates in some regions. This has resulted in the re-emergence of diseases like **measles**, which had been largely eliminated in high-income countries.

Another challenge is **logistics** in reaching remote or conflict-ridden areas. In low-income countries, **poor infrastructure**, **lack of healthcare personnel**, and **difficult terrain** make it challenging to deliver vaccines to those in need. In some areas, vaccine storage is difficult due to the lack of **cold chain systems**, which are necessary to keep vaccines at the correct temperature until they are administered.

Political instability and conflict also hinder vaccination efforts. In regions affected by war or political unrest, vaccination teams often face security risks, and the breakdown of health infrastructure can lead to low vaccination coverage. This creates pockets of vulnerability where diseases can spread and potentially re-emerge on a larger scale.

The Future of Vaccination and Disease Control

Recent advances in vaccine technology, such as **mRNA vaccines**, are opening new possibilities for preventing and controlling infectious diseases. The rapid development of **COVID-19 vaccines** using mRNA technology demonstrated the potential for faster and more flexible vaccine production. This technology can be adapted quickly to target emerging diseases, offering promise for future vaccination programs.

Efforts to eradicate diseases like **measles, rubella**, and **polio** continue, and new vaccines are being developed for diseases such as **malaria** and **HIV**. Expanding global access to vaccines through initiatives like **Gavi, the Vaccine Alliance**, is essential for ensuring that low- and middle-income countries benefit from these advances. Addressing challenges like vaccine hesitancy, infrastructure limitations, and political barriers will be critical to the future success of global vaccination efforts.

CHAPTER 16: FUTURE TRENDS AND CHALLENGES IN EPIDEMIOLOGY

Big Data and Epidemiology: Opportunities and Challenges

Big data is opening new avenues for understanding disease patterns, predicting outbreaks, and shaping public health interventions. Big data refers to extremely large datasets that can be analyzed computationally to reveal trends, associations, and patterns. With the increasing availability of health data from diverse sources—ranging from **electronic health records (EHRs)** to **social media** and **genomics**—epidemiologists have unprecedented tools to study health at both the population and individual levels. However, alongside these opportunities come significant challenges related to data management, privacy, and the need for appropriate analytical methods.

Opportunities in Big Data for Epidemiology

Real-time monitoring is one of the most significant opportunities big data offers to epidemiology. Traditional epidemiologic methods often rely on data that is collected retrospectively, meaning there is a delay between the onset of an outbreak and the identification of the pattern. In contrast, big data, sourced from **EHRs**, **social media posts**, **search engine queries**, and even **wearable devices**, allows for **real-time disease surveillance**. This kind of data can help detect emerging outbreaks early and allows public health officials to intervene more quickly.

For example, platforms like **Google Flu Trends** tried to use search queries to estimate flu activity in real-time. While it faced limitations, the approach highlighted the potential of using non-traditional data sources for disease surveillance. Real-time data from sources like **social media** can be useful for tracking outbreaks, especially when combined with traditional surveillance methods.

Another opportunity big data brings is **predictive modeling**. By analyzing massive datasets, epidemiologists can identify **patterns** and **risk factors** that may not be apparent in smaller studies. Predictive models built from big data can help estimate the likelihood of disease outbreaks, as well as forecast the progression of diseases based on historical and real-time information. For example, analyzing hospital admissions and climate data can help predict the **seasonality of diseases** like malaria or influenza. These insights allow public health officials to allocate resources more efficiently, such as stockpiling vaccines or deploying healthcare workers to high-risk areas before an outbreak peaks.

Genomic data is another powerful component of big data in epidemiology. With the **sequencing of the human genome** and the growing field of **genomics**, researchers can now study how genetic variations influence disease susceptibility and transmission. For example, during the **COVID-19 pandemic**, genomic data was critical in tracking the evolution of the virus, identifying new variants, and understanding how these variants spread across populations. This ability to quickly sequence and analyze pathogen genomes is revolutionizing the way public health responds to infectious diseases.

Big data also offers opportunities for **personalized medicine**. By combining data from **biometrics**, **genomics**, and **environmental factors**, epidemiologists can help tailor public health interventions to specific populations. For example, big data can help identify which individuals or groups might respond better to certain treatments or preventive measures based on their genetic profiles or other risk factors.

Challenges in Using Big Data

Despite its potential, big data in epidemiology comes with significant challenges. One of the foremost issues is **data quality**. Not all big data sources are created equal, and much of the information collected from social media, search engines, or even wearable devices can be **incomplete**, **inaccurate**, or **biased**. For example, social media data may reflect the experiences and behaviors of certain demographics more than others, leading to skewed insights. Therefore, ensuring the **reliability** and **representativeness** of the data is a major hurdle for epidemiologists.

Another challenge is **data integration**. Health data comes from various sources— **EHRs**, **clinical trials**, **laboratories**, **genomics databases**, and **public health registries**. These datasets often use different formats and standards, making it difficult to combine them into a cohesive whole. Standardizing data collection methods and creating interoperable systems are critical for making full use of big data in epidemiology. Otherwise, insights drawn from fragmented or poorly integrated data may be misleading.

Privacy and ethical concerns are also significant challenges in the use of big data for public health. Health data, especially when linked to individual records, is highly sensitive. The more comprehensive and detailed the dataset, the greater the risk of breaching **patient confidentiality**. As more health information becomes digitized and shared across systems, it becomes increasingly important to balance the need for comprehensive data with the protection of individual privacy. **De-identification** of data—removing personally identifiable information—can mitigate this risk, but it's not foolproof, as advances in data analytics can sometimes re-identify individuals even in anonymized datasets.

There is also the issue of **data overload**. Big data can produce enormous quantities of information, making it difficult for epidemiologists to sift through and identify what is truly meaningful. **Advanced analytical tools**, such as **machine learning** and **artificial intelligence (AI)**, are needed to process and analyze these massive datasets. However, these tools come with their own set of challenges, such as the **black-box problem**, where the algorithm's decision-making process is opaque, making it difficult to interpret the results or trust the insights.

Equity is another challenge. As big data becomes increasingly central to public health, there is a risk that populations with less access to digital technology—such as those in low-income regions or rural areas—will be underrepresented in datasets. This can lead to biased findings that overlook the health needs of these communities. Ensuring that data collection efforts are inclusive and that interventions are equitable across all populations is critical to preventing further health disparities.

The Role of Artificial Intelligence in Disease Surveillance

Artificial intelligence (AI) is transforming **disease surveillance**, offering new ways to detect, predict, and respond to outbreaks of infectious diseases. By automating data analysis and recognizing patterns across vast datasets, AI can help public health officials identify potential threats more quickly and accurately. In a world where new diseases can spread globally in days, AI offers a powerful technology for real-time monitoring and early detection of outbreaks.

Early Detection and Real-Time Monitoring

AI can process enormous amounts of data far faster than humans, allowing for **real-time disease surveillance**. Traditional disease surveillance systems often rely on manual reporting and data analysis, which can lead to delays in detecting outbreaks. AI systems, on the other hand, can analyze data from multiple sources—including **electronic health records (EHRs)**, **social media**, and **news reports**—to identify unusual patterns that may signal the start of an outbreak.

For example, AI platforms like **BlueDot** and **HealthMap** use natural language processing (NLP) to scan news articles, public health reports, and social media for signs of emerging health threats. **BlueDot**, in particular, was able to detect the early signs of the **COVID-19 outbreak** days before official health organizations issued public warnings, demonstrating how AI can enhance early detection. By spotting disease patterns quickly, AI can give public health officials a head start in responding to potential outbreaks.

Predictive Modeling

AI is also revolutionizing **predictive modeling**, which uses data to forecast how diseases will spread. Traditional epidemiological models rely on fixed parameters, such as **transmission rates** and **population density**, to predict how a disease will behave. While effective, these models often struggle to account for complex variables like human behavior, climate changes, or mobility patterns.

AI can overcome these limitations by learning from **real-time data** and adjusting predictions as new information comes in. For example, during the COVID-19 pandemic, AI models were used to predict the spread of the virus based on factors such as **population movement**, **mask usage**, and **social distancing practices**. These AI-driven models provided more flexible and accurate predictions, helping governments and health organizations allocate resources like **ventilators**, **hospital beds**, and **vaccines** more effectively.

In addition, AI can integrate data from **genomic sequencing** to track the evolution of pathogens, helping scientists anticipate which **mutations** might lead to more infectious or deadly strains. This was critical during the emergence of the **Delta** and **Omicron variants** of SARS-CoV-2, where real-time genomic analysis helped adjust public health strategies.

Automation and Efficiency

One of AI's greatest strengths is its ability to **automate tasks**, reducing the burden on human workers. AI can automate the collection and analysis of data from various sources, providing a constant stream of updated information without the need for manual input. This allows public health agencies to monitor disease trends more efficiently and frees up human workers to focus on tasks that require critical thinking and decision-making.

For instance, AI can automatically scan laboratory test results and hospital admissions to detect patterns that may suggest an outbreak of **foodborne illness** or other diseases. By flagging these patterns early, AI can trigger investigations before the outbreak spreads more widely.

Overcoming Data Gaps and Bias

While AI offers many advantages, it is not without challenges. One significant issue is **data bias**. AI systems are only as good as the data they are trained on. If certain populations—such as rural or low-income communities—are underrepresented in the data, AI models may fail to detect outbreaks in these areas or may produce biased predictions that overlook their specific needs.

To address this, it is crucial to ensure that data used in AI models is representative of all populations and regions. This may involve improving **data collection** in underserved areas, as well as ensuring that AI algorithms are designed to minimize bias. Ethical considerations also come into play, especially when AI is used to track individual health data. Privacy concerns must be carefully managed to protect patient information while still allowing for effective disease surveillance.

Future of AI in Disease Surveillance

Looking ahead, AI will likely have an even greater role in **pandemic preparedness** and **response**. As AI technologies improve, they will become more adept at analyzing complex variables, such as how **climate change**, **migration**, and **urbanization** affect the spread of diseases. In addition, AI could be integrated with **wearable health devices** to monitor individual health in real-time, flagging potential symptoms of infectious diseases before individuals even seek medical attention.

AI's ability to process and learn from vast amounts of data offers a potential way to control infectious diseases. By improving early detection, enhancing predictive modeling, and automating surveillance tasks, AI has the potential to revolutionize public health and prevent future pandemics from reaching the scale of COVID-19.

Climate Change and Its Impact on Disease Patterns

Climate change is reshaping the world's ecosystems, and with these changes come significant impacts on **disease patterns**. As global temperatures rise, weather patterns shift, and extreme weather events become more frequent, the geographic distribution and seasonal activity of many infectious diseases are changing. This shift poses new challenges for public health systems around the world, as diseases that were once confined to certain regions or seasons are now appearing in new areas.

Vector-Borne Diseases

One of the most significant impacts of climate change is the changing distribution of **vector-borne diseases**—those transmitted by insects such as mosquitoes, ticks, and fleas. Diseases like **malaria**, **dengue fever**, **Zika virus**, and **Lyme disease** are highly sensitive to environmental conditions, particularly temperature and rainfall patterns.

Mosquitoes, which transmit malaria and dengue fever, thrive in warmer, wetter climates. As global temperatures rise, these insects are expanding their habitats into previously cooler regions, bringing diseases with them. For instance, the range of the **Aedes mosquito**, which spreads dengue, is increasing in areas that were once too cold to sustain these insects, including parts of **Europe** and **North America**. This has led to the spread of **dengue fever** into areas where it was not previously endemic.

Similarly, **Lyme disease**, transmitted by **ticks**, is also spreading as climate change extends the range of these vectors into more northern latitudes. Warmer temperatures are leading to longer tick seasons, allowing the bacteria that cause Lyme disease to infect more people over an extended period.

Waterborne Diseases and Flooding

Climate change is also affecting the spread of **waterborne diseases**, particularly in areas that experience increased rainfall and flooding. Diseases like **cholera** and **cryptosporidiosis** spread through contaminated water, and heavy rains or floods can contaminate drinking water supplies with pathogens. As flooding becomes more frequent and severe due to climate change, the risk of waterborne disease outbreaks increases, particularly in areas with poor sanitation infrastructure.

In coastal regions, rising sea levels are contributing to the **salinization of freshwater** supplies, complicating water access and sanitation efforts. Additionally, warmer water temperatures can promote the growth of harmful bacteria and algae, increasing the risk of diseases like **Vibrio infections** and harmful algal blooms.

Changes in Disease Seasonality

Climate change is also affecting the **seasonality** of diseases, with some infections becoming more prevalent at times of the year when they were previously rare. For example, **influenza** outbreaks typically occur in winter in temperate regions, but as temperatures rise, the seasonal boundaries of flu activity may shift. This complicates efforts to predict and prepare for outbreaks, especially in regions that are unaccustomed to dealing with the disease during certain times of the year.

The **El Niño** and **La Niña** phenomena, which are influenced by climate change, also impact disease seasonality by altering rainfall patterns and temperatures in different parts of the world. In regions affected by El Niño, increased rainfall can lead to spikes in diseases like **malaria** and **dengue**, while droughts associated with La Niña can reduce the prevalence of certain diseases but increase others, such as those related to food and water shortages.

Food Security and Nutrition

Climate change is affecting **food security**, which in turn influences disease patterns. **Droughts, heatwaves,** and **changing growing seasons** are reducing crop yields in many parts of the world, leading to malnutrition, particularly in low-income regions. Malnutrition weakens the immune system, making individuals more vulnerable to infectious diseases. In some areas, climate change is also affecting the **nutritional content** of staple crops, further exacerbating health problems related to diet.

In regions where agriculture is a primary source of livelihood, the disruption caused by climate change can force communities to migrate, increasing the spread of diseases. **Displacement** due to drought, rising sea levels, or other climate-related factors often leads to overcrowded living conditions with poor sanitation, creating environments ripe for outbreaks of infectious diseases.

Preparing for Future Disease Patterns

The impacts of climate change on disease patterns are already being felt, but they will likely worsen in the coming decades. Public health systems must adapt to these new realities by improving **surveillance, vector control,** and **water sanitation infrastructure**. Early warning systems that monitor environmental changes, such as temperature shifts and rainfall patterns, can help predict disease outbreaks and allow for timely public health interventions.

International cooperation will be critical to addressing the global nature of these challenges. As diseases spread across borders due to climate change, countries must collaborate on solutions, share data, and coordinate responses. By understanding the links between climate change and disease patterns, public health officials can better prepare for the changing landscape of global health.

CHAPTER 17: HISTORY AND TERMS

History of Epidemiology

Here we cover the history of epidemiology in a timeline format, covering key events and developments over the centuries.

Ancient and Early Foundations (Circa 400 BCE - 1500 CE)

400 BCE - Hippocrates Proposes the Environmental Theory of Disease

Hippocrates, often called the "Father of Medicine," was among the first to suggest that diseases might be linked to environmental factors, behavior, and diet, rather than being punishments from the gods. In his work *On Airs, Waters, and Places*, Hippocrates emphasized that air, water quality, and living conditions might influence health. Although his theories lacked scientific evidence, they laid the foundation for the idea that external factors contribute to illness, a core concept in epidemiology.

14th Century - The Black Death (1347-1351)

One of the deadliest pandemics in human history, the Black Death (caused by the bacterium *Yersinia pestis*) swept through Europe, killing an estimated 25-30 million people. The plague triggered some of the earliest epidemiological responses. Officials in cities like Venice and Milan established quarantine stations to isolate the sick, one of the first attempts at public health measures based on observational epidemiology. Although the nature of disease was not understood, these efforts marked a step toward disease control through population-level interventions.

The Early Modern Period (1500-1800)

1662 - John Graunt and the Birth of Vital Statistics

John Graunt, a London haberdasher, is considered one of the first demographers and epidemiologists. He systematically collected and analyzed mortality data, publishing his findings in *Natural and Political Observations Made upon the Bills of Mortality*. By reviewing death records, he identified patterns of mortality and morbidity, including seasonal variations in deaths and differences between urban and rural areas. His work laid the groundwork for statistical methods in epidemiology, offering early insights into how diseases affect populations.

1700 - Bernardino Ramazzini and Occupational Health

Bernardino Ramazzini, an Italian physician, is often referred to as the "Father of Occupational Medicine." In his book *De Morbis Artificum Diatriba* (Diseases of Workers), he detailed the relationship between various occupations and diseases. He identified hazards in workers' environments and advocated for improved working conditions to prevent illness, an important development in the epidemiological study of environmental and occupational factors affecting health.

1796 - Edward Jenner and the First Vaccine

Edward Jenner, an English physician, performed one of the most famous experiments in medical history when he vaccinated a young boy, James Phipps, against smallpox using cowpox material. His work demonstrated that exposure to a mild disease could provide immunity to a more severe one, sparking the birth of vaccination and preventive medicine. This was a turning point in epidemiology, demonstrating the importance of understanding disease transmission and developing population-level interventions to control diseases.

The 19th Century: The Birth of Modern Epidemiology

1854 - John Snow and the Cholera Outbreak

Often hailed as the "Father of Modern Epidemiology," John Snow made a groundbreaking contribution to the field during the cholera outbreak in London in 1854. Snow suspected that cholera was transmitted through contaminated water rather than miasma (the then-dominant theory of disease transmission). He mapped the cases of cholera around a specific water pump on Broad Street and convinced officials to remove the pump handle, which led to a decrease in cases. This was one of the first examples of using epidemiological methods (mapping and case studies) to identify the source of an outbreak and implement public health interventions.

1850s - Florence Nightingale and Hospital Sanitation

Florence Nightingale, a British nurse and statistician, revolutionized hospital care during the Crimean War. Through her detailed records and statistical analysis, she demonstrated that poor sanitary conditions in hospitals contributed to high mortality rates. Nightingale's use of data to drive changes in health practices is considered a key contribution to epidemiology and public health, emphasizing the importance of environment and sanitation in disease prevention.

1876 - Robert Koch and Germ Theory

Robert Koch, a German physician, confirmed the germ theory of disease when he identified *Bacillus anthracis* as the bacterium that causes anthrax. His work with infectious diseases, including tuberculosis and cholera, helped establish microbiology as a cornerstone of epidemiology. Koch developed a set of postulates (Koch's postulates) that provided a framework for linking specific pathogens to specific diseases, laying the foundation for modern epidemiology's focus on disease causation.

Early 20th Century: The Expansion of Epidemiology

1918 - The Spanish Flu Pandemic

The Spanish Flu pandemic of 1918-1919 was one of the deadliest in history, killing an estimated 50 million people worldwide. This global pandemic spurred advances in public health systems and highlighted the need for international collaboration in epidemiology. It also emphasized the importance of tracking and analyzing disease patterns to predict outbreaks and guide public health interventions, leading to the development of global surveillance systems.

1920s - Sydenstricker and Population Health Surveys

Edgar Sydenstricker was a pioneer in the use of population health surveys to gather data on public health. His surveys during the 1920s aimed to collect comprehensive health data on different segments of the population, particularly during the Great Depression. His work contributed to the development of surveillance systems and the study of social determinants of health, emphasizing that economic and social conditions greatly affect public health outcomes.

1930s - The Framingham Heart Study (Began 1948)

The Framingham Heart Study, which began in the late 1940s, was one of the first large-scale epidemiological studies to investigate chronic diseases, specifically cardiovascular disease. Researchers followed a cohort of individuals over several decades to study the risk factors associated with heart disease. The study introduced the concept of "risk factors" into the field of epidemiology, shifting the focus from infectious diseases to chronic, non-communicable diseases.

Mid-20th Century: Expanding Methods and Scope

1950 - Doll and Hill's Study on Smoking and Lung Cancer

Sir Richard Doll and Austin Bradford Hill conducted one of the first epidemiological studies linking smoking to lung cancer. Their work, which began in the 1950s, involved case-control and cohort studies that provided compelling evidence of the harmful effects of smoking. This research was crucial in shifting public health policy and launching anti-smoking campaigns, demonstrating the power of epidemiological studies to influence policy and behavioral change.

1959 - The World Health Organization (WHO) Expands Global Health Monitoring

The WHO established global surveillance systems for monitoring infectious diseases, such as polio and smallpox, which enabled better responses to international outbreaks. This marked a significant expansion in the role of epidemiology in global health and led to the eventual eradication of smallpox in 1980, thanks to coordinated vaccination campaigns.

Late 20th Century: The Rise of Modern Epidemiology

1970s - Epidemiology of Chronic Diseases

By the 1970s, epidemiology had shifted its focus beyond infectious diseases to include chronic diseases such as cancer, heart disease, and diabetes. The use of large-scale cohort studies, such as the Nurses' Health Study and the British Doctors' Study, expanded the understanding of risk factors associated with lifestyle and environmental exposures, paving the way for prevention strategies.

1981 - HIV/AIDS Epidemic and Global Health

The first cases of AIDS were reported in 1981, and the epidemic that followed highlighted the importance of epidemiological surveillance, rapid data collection, and response to emerging health crises. The global effort to track and control the spread of HIV/AIDS showcased how epidemiology could be used to address new and rapidly evolving health threats. It also emphasized the need for public health education and behavioral interventions.

1980s-1990s - Advances in Molecular and Genetic Epidemiology

The rise of molecular biology and genetics in the 1980s and 1990s allowed epidemiologists to study diseases at the genetic level. Researchers began to investigate the role of genetic factors in diseases, particularly cancer, cardiovascular disease, and diabetes. The combination of traditional epidemiological methods with molecular biology techniques has given rise to modern genetic epidemiology, which explores the complex interactions between genes and the environment in disease causation.

21st Century: Big Data and Global Health Challenges

2003 - SARS Outbreak and Global Surveillance

The 2003 outbreak of Severe Acute Respiratory Syndrome (SARS) highlighted the importance of international collaboration and global health surveillance. Rapid epidemiological investigations and sharing of information between countries helped control the outbreak, demonstrating the need for real-time data sharing and global communication systems in the modern era.

2014-2016 - Ebola Outbreak in West Africa

The Ebola outbreak in West Africa between 2014 and 2016 was one of the deadliest in history, with over 11,000 deaths. The global response, including the use of epidemiological surveillance, contact tracing, and quarantine measures, showed how epidemiological tools could be adapted to emerging and high-risk health threats in complex and resource-poor settings.

2020 - COVID-19 Pandemic

The COVID-19 pandemic marks one of the most significant public health crises in recent history. Epidemiological modeling, contact tracing, and global surveillance systems were crucial in tracking the spread of the virus, understanding risk factors, and guiding policy decisions. The pandemic also showcased the increasing role of **big data** and **artificial intelligence** in real-time disease tracking and prediction. Epidemiologists worldwide used data from mobile apps, social media, and public health records to monitor infection rates, predict outbreaks, and assess the effectiveness of interventions like social distancing and vaccines. The pandemic highlighted both the power and the challenges of modern epidemiology, particularly in coordinating global responses and addressing misinformation.

Big Data and Epidemiology (Ongoing)

The rise of big data and advanced computational methods has transformed epidemiology in the 21st century. Epidemiologists now have access to vast amounts of health data from various sources, including electronic medical records, wearable devices, and social media. This wealth of information allows for more precise modeling and prediction of disease outbreaks, the identification of trends in chronic disease, and the development of personalized public health interventions.

Machine learning and artificial intelligence (AI) are also increasingly being integrated into epidemiological practices. These tools can process large datasets more quickly and efficiently than traditional methods, enabling more accurate predictions of disease spread and potential outbreaks. AI-powered models are now used to optimize vaccine distribution, predict high-risk populations for chronic diseases, and detect new patterns in emerging infectious diseases.

Climate Change and Health

As the 21st century progresses, the impact of climate change on global health has become a growing focus for epidemiologists. Climate change influences the spread of infectious diseases, particularly those transmitted by vectors like mosquitoes (e.g., malaria and dengue fever). It also contributes to the frequency and severity of extreme weather events, such as heatwaves and floods, which pose direct and indirect risks to population health.

Epidemiologists are increasingly studying how environmental changes affect disease patterns and are working to develop predictive models to mitigate the health impacts of climate change. This has become a new frontier in global health, with public health officials relying on epidemiological data to prepare for and respond to these emerging health threats.

Terms and Definitions

These definitions provide a solid foundation in understanding epidemiological concepts and terms commonly used in research, public health practice, and disease control.

- **Epidemiology**: The study of the distribution and determinants of health-related states or events in specified populations, and the application of this study to control health problems.
- **Incidence**: The number of new cases of a disease or condition in a specific population during a defined time period.

- **Prevalence**: The total number of cases (new and existing) of a disease in a population at a given time.
- **Morbidity**: The presence of illness or disease within a population.
- **Mortality**: The occurrence of death within a population.
- **Risk Factor**: An attribute, characteristic, or exposure that increases the likelihood of developing a disease or injury.
- **Relative Risk (RR)**: The ratio of the probability of an event occurring in an exposed group to the probability of it occurring in a non-exposed group.
- **Odds Ratio (OR)**: A measure of association between exposure and outcome, comparing the odds of the event occurring in the exposed group to the odds in the non-exposed group.
- **Cohort Study**: A longitudinal study that follows a group of people (cohort) over time to assess the incidence of disease and its relation to suspected risk factors.
- **Case-Control Study**: An observational study that compares individuals with a specific condition (cases) to those without the condition (controls) to identify factors that might contribute to the condition.
- **Cross-Sectional Study**: A type of observational study that analyzes data from a population at a specific point in time.
- **Longitudinal Study**: A study that follows the same group of individuals over a period of time to observe changes and developments.
- **Bias**: A systematic error that leads to an incorrect estimate of the association between exposure and outcome.
- **Selection Bias**: Bias introduced when the participants selected for a study are not representative of the target population.
- **Information Bias**: Bias that occurs when the measurement of exposure, outcome, or both is inaccurate.
- **Recall Bias**: A type of information bias that occurs when participants do not accurately remember or report past events or exposures.
- **Confounding**: A situation in which a third variable influences both the exposure and the outcome, distorting the apparent relationship between them.
- **Effect Modification**: A situation where the effect of the main exposure on the outcome differs depending on the level of another variable.
- **Epidemic**: An outbreak of disease that occurs at a higher frequency than normal in a specific population or area.
- **Pandemic**: An epidemic that spreads across countries or continents, affecting a large number of people globally.
- **Endemic**: The constant presence of a disease or condition in a particular geographic area or population.
- **Herd Immunity**: The resistance to the spread of an infectious disease within a population that results if a sufficiently high proportion of individuals are immune to the disease.
- **Quarantine**: The separation and restriction of movement of people who may have been exposed to a contagious disease but are not yet symptomatic.
- **Incubation Period**: The period between exposure to an infectious agent and the onset of symptoms.
- **Outbreak**: A sudden increase in the number of cases of a disease above what is normally expected in a localized area.
- **Zoonosis**: A disease that can be transmitted from animals to humans.

- **Nosocomial Infection**: An infection that is acquired in a hospital or healthcare setting.
- **Index Case**: The first identified case of a disease in an outbreak.
- **Attack Rate**: The proportion of exposed individuals who become ill during an outbreak.
- **Case Fatality Rate (CFR)**: The proportion of people who die from a specific disease among all individuals diagnosed with the disease.
- **Incidence Rate**: The rate at which new cases of a disease occur in a population over a specific period of time.
- **Person-Time**: A measurement that accounts for the number of individuals in a study and the amount of time each individual spends in the study.
- **Cumulative Incidence**: The proportion of a population that develops a condition over a specific time period.
- **Relative Risk Reduction (RRR)**: The percentage reduction in risk in the exposed group compared to the non-exposed group.
- **Attributable Risk (AR)**: The difference in the risk of a condition between exposed and non-exposed individuals.
- **Number Needed to Treat (NNT)**: The number of people who need to receive a treatment to prevent one additional adverse outcome.
- **Number Needed to Harm (NNH)**: The number of people who need to be exposed to a risk factor to cause one additional harmful outcome.
- **Primary Prevention**: Measures aimed at preventing the onset of disease (e.g., vaccinations, healthy lifestyle promotion).
- **Secondary Prevention**: Measures aimed at detecting and treating diseases early (e.g., screening programs).
- **Tertiary Prevention**: Measures aimed at reducing the impact of long-term illness or injury (e.g., rehabilitation programs).
- **Surveillance**: The continuous, systematic collection, analysis, and interpretation of health-related data needed for the planning, implementation, and evaluation of public health practice.
- **Sentinel Surveillance**: Monitoring of disease trends in specific populations or institutions to detect outbreaks or emerging trends.
- **Vital Statistics**: The collection and analysis of data related to births, deaths, marriages, and other life events.
- **Ecological Study**: A study in which the units of analysis are populations or groups of people rather than individuals.
- **Cluster**: A group of cases of a disease or condition that occur closely together in time or location.
- **Randomized Controlled Trial (RCT)**: An experimental study in which participants are randomly assigned to treatment or control groups to evaluate the effectiveness of an intervention.
- **Blinding**: A technique used in clinical trials to prevent bias, where participants and/or investigators do not know which group participants are in (treatment or control).
- **Double-Blind Study**: A study in which neither the participants nor the investigators know who is receiving the treatment or placebo.
- **Placebo**: An inactive substance or treatment given to a control group in a clinical trial to assess the true effect of the intervention being tested.

- **Cohort**: A group of individuals who share a common characteristic or experience within a defined period.
- **Prospective Study**: A study that follows participants forward in time to observe outcomes.
- **Retrospective Study**: A study that looks back at past events to determine the cause of a current outcome.
- **Latency Period**: The time between exposure to a risk factor and the manifestation of a disease.
- **Exposure**: Any factor (e.g., behavior, environmental condition, biological agent) that may influence the risk of developing a disease or health outcome.
- **Dose-Response Relationship**: The relationship between the amount of exposure to a factor and the risk of developing a health outcome.
- **Confounding Variable**: A variable that influences both the independent variable (exposure) and the dependent variable (outcome), potentially distorting the association between the two.
- **Survival Rate**: The proportion of people in a study or treatment group who are still alive for a certain period of time after diagnosis or treatment.
- **Validity**: The degree to which a measurement or study accurately reflects or assesses the concept being investigated.
- **Reliability**: The consistency of a measure or study; the extent to which results can be reproduced under the same conditions.
- **Sensitivity**: The ability of a test to correctly identify those who have a disease (true positives).
- **Specificity**: The ability of a test to correctly identify those who do not have a disease (true negatives).
- **Positive Predictive Value (PPV)**: The probability that individuals with a positive test result truly have the disease.
- **Negative Predictive Value (NPV)**: The probability that individuals with a negative test result truly do not have the disease.
- **Public Health Surveillance**: The continuous monitoring of diseases, injuries, or health risks in populations for the purpose of control and prevention.
- **Incidental Findings**: Unexpected discoveries made during the course of epidemiological research or clinical testing.
- **Epidemiologic Transition**: A shift in disease patterns in a population, from infectious diseases being the primary cause of death to chronic, non-communicable diseases becoming dominant.

AFTERWORD

Thank you for joining me on this overview of the field of epidemiology. I hope that as you've worked your way through the chapters, you've gained a solid understanding of the science behind disease tracking and control. Epidemiology is a field that combines curiosity, data, and a genuine desire to improve public health. It's not just about analyzing numbers or conducting studies—it's about making a real difference in the lives of individuals and communities.

Whether you are new to epidemiology or already familiar with its concepts, I hope this book has provided clarity and insight. From understanding the fundamentals of disease frequency and study designs to tackling more advanced topics like genetic epidemiology and global health, you now have the concepts and frameworks to think like an epidemiologist. You've learned how data shapes public health decisions, how outbreaks are investigated, and how we identify the causes of both infectious and chronic diseases.

The beauty of epidemiology lies in its practical applications. The principles you've learned here aren't confined to textbooks or academic discussions—they are used every day by public health professionals to protect people's health. From tracking flu outbreaks to identifying cancer risk factors, epidemiologists are at the forefront of keeping populations healthy and responding to health crises.

As you continue your own path in this field—whether as a student, professional, or simply someone interested in public health—remember that epidemiology is always evolving. New diseases emerge, new technologies develop, and the global landscape continues to change. Staying curious and keeping an eye on current trends will help you remain engaged and informed in this continuously changing field.

One key lesson from epidemiology is that health is a collective effort. The patterns of disease that we study reflect larger social, environmental, and behavioral factors. No single discipline can solve these issues alone, and collaboration is critical. Whether you work in public health, healthcare, or another related field, your role contributes to the larger goal of improving health outcomes.

As we look to the future, epidemiology will remain essential in addressing public health challenges, from pandemics to chronic diseases and climate-related health risks. I hope this book has inspired you to continue learning and engaging with these important issues. Thank you for taking the time to explore this fascinating field with me, and I wish you all the best in your continued journey of understanding and applying epidemiology to make a positive impact on the world.

Stay curious, stay engaged, and remember that even small steps in public health can lead to big changes.

Made in the USA
Columbia, SC
30 November 2024

1d394f6d-d0ea-4567-8d8e-7cd3836040e5R01